Multi-professional Learning for Nurses

Nurse Education in Practice Series

Multi-professional Learning for Nurses: Breaking the boundaries
Edited by Sally Glen and Tony Leiba

Problem-based Learning in Nursing: A new model for a new context?
Edited by Sally Glen and Kay Wilkie

Clinical Skills in Nursing: The return of the practical room?
Edited by Maggie Nicol and Sally Glen

Nurse Education in Practice Series
Series Standing Order
ISBN 0-333-98590-7
(outside North America only)

You can receive future titles in this series as they are published by placing a standing order. Please contact your bookseller or, in the case of difficulty, write to us at the address below with your name and address, the title of the series and the ISBN quoted above.

Customer Services Department, Macmillan Distribution Ltd
Houndmills, Basingstoke, Hampshire RG21 6XS, England

Multi-professional Learning for Nurses

Breaking the boundaries

Edited by

Sally Glen
and
Tony Leiba

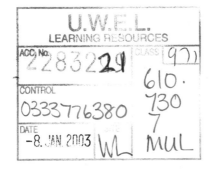
palgrave

First published 2002 by
PALGRAVE
Houndmills, Basingstoke, Hampshire RG21 6XS and
175 Fifth Avenue, New York, N.Y. 10010
Companies and representatives throughout the world

PALGRAVE is the new global academic imprint of
St. Martin's Press LLC Scholarly and Reference Division and
Palgrave Publishers Ltd (formerly Macmillan Press Ltd).

ISBN 0–333–77638–0

10 9 8 7 6 5 4 3 2 1
11 10 09 08 07 06 05 04 03 02

Printed in Malaysia

Contents

List of Figures and Table   viii
List of Contributors   ix
Foreword   xi
Preface   xiii

1 The Context – Why the Current Interest?   1
    Stuart Cable
    Introduction   1
    Multi-professionalism in policy   2
    Multi-professionalism in education   7
    Multi-professionalism in practice   15
    Conclusion   19
    Note   20
    References   20

**2 Multi-professional Education: Definitions and
    Perspectives**   25
    Tony Leiba
    Defining terms   26
    Opportunities for multi-professional education   28
    Multi-professional assumptions   29
    Theories of multi-professional education   32
    Multi-professional education and the future   34
    References   36

3 Joint Training for Integrated Care   40
    Dave Sims
    Introduction   40
    Historical context   42
    Local demand for joint training   43
    The rationale for joint training   44
    The structure of the programme   45
    A framework of common competencies   47
    Inter-professional competence   48
    A programme based on partnership   50

Challenges encountered   51
Programme evaluation   53
Lessons learned from the previous programmes   54
Evaluation of the South Bank programme   55
Conclusion   58
References   59

4 **Inter-professional Teaching Programme on Normal
   Labour for Midwifery and Medical Students   61**
   Margaret McCarey and Gary Mires
   Introduction   61
   Context   62
   The initiative   64
   Teaching/Learning methods   65
   Planning of the programme   67
   Delivery of the programme   67
   Evaluation process   70
   Evaluation results   71
   Limitations   74
   Keys to success   75
   Implications for the future   76
   Conclusion   76
   References   77
   Appendix 1   78
   Appendix 2   82

5 **Learning Clinical Skills: an Inter-professional
   Approach   84**
   Maggie Nicol and Mark Chaput de Saintonge
   Introduction   84
   Inter-professional clinical skills programme   86
   The programme structure   87
   Discussion   91
   Clinical governance   92
   References   95

6 **A Perspective of Shared Teaching in Ethics   97**
   Cecilia Edward, Ann Roberts and June Small
   Introduction   97
   The key   98

The ideal   98
The picture   101
Aims and learning outcomes   102
Educational strategy   104
Learning and teaching tools   105
Reality challenges   106
Conclusion to reality   109
Evaluation   110
Conclusion   110
References   111
Appendix   112

7   Evaluation of an Inter-professional Training Ward:
    Pilot Phase   116
    Della Freeth and Scott Reeves
    Introduction   116
    The inter-professional training ward, London   117
    Evaluation   118
    Discussion of evaluation findings   119
    Conclusions   133
    Glossary   136
    Acknowledgements   136
    References   136

8   Inter-professional Education: the Way Forward 139
    Sally Glen
    Introduction   139
    Multiple stakeholder perspectives   140
    An integrated approach to care   141
    A system sympathetic to innovation   143
    An evidence-based agenda   145
    Conclusion   146
    References   146

Index   148

List of Figures and Table

Figures

1.1 The Clyde Report: a failure of multi-professional
    function and recommendations for action   4
1.2 Creating contact between students: a rationale for
    multi-professional education   14
1.3 Hospital practice: the causes of conflict in the
    medical and nursing teams   17
3.1 The integration of learning outcomes into one
    common competency framework   48
3.2 The common competency framework   49
4.1 Assigned responsibility for clinical tasks
    (Section A) – all students ($p < 0.001$: chi squared
    439.5 pre versus post course)   72
4.2 Assigned responsibility for information provision
    (Section B) – all students ($p < 0.001$: chi squared
    245.74 pre versus post course)   73
5.1 Clinical Scenarios used in the inter-professional
    study   88
6.1 Sample case studies/statements   105

Table

1.1 Aims of inter-disciplinarity   10

List of Contributors

Stuart Cable Lecturer in Nursing, School of Nursing and Midwifery, University of Dundee, Scotland.

Mark Chaput de Saintonge Director of Clinical Skills and Consultant Physician, St Bartholomew's and the London School of Medicine and Dentistry, London, England.

Cecilia Edward Nursing Lecturer, School of Nursing and Midwifery, University of Dundee, Scotland.

Della Freeth Senior Lecturer – Research at Clinical Skills, St Bartholomew School of Nursing and Midwifery, City University, London, England.

Sally Glen Dean, Professor of Nursing Education, St Bartholomew's School of Nursing and Midwifery, City University, London, England.

Tony Leiba Lecturer, St Bartholomew's School of Nursing and Midwifery, City University, London, England.

Margaret McCarey Senior Midwifery Lecturer, School of Nursing and Midwifery, University of Dundee, Scotland.

Gary Miers Senior Lecturer and Consultant Obstetrician and Gynaecology, School of Medicine, University of Dundee, Ninewells Hospital and Medical School, Dundee, Scotland.

Maggie Nicol Senior Lecturer in Clinical Skills, St Bartholomew's School of Nursing and Midwifery, City University, London, England.

Scott Reeves Research Officer, St Bartholomew School of Nursing and Midwifery, City University, London, England.

Dave Sims Principal Lecturer, Faculty of Health, South Bank University, London, England.

June Small Midwifery Lecturer, School of Nursing and Midwifery, University of Dundee, Scotland.

Ann Roberts Nursing Lecturer, School of Nursing and Midwifery, University of Dundee, Scotland.

Foreword

Seldom has publication of a book been so timely as the NHS National Plan accords nurses more responsibilities and more opportunities for career progression, and they work with others to create more flexible services in response to the expressed needs and expectations of patients (Secretary of State for Health, 2000).

Inter-professional education is once again being invoked to engender support from the health professions to implement new policies in a spirit of give and take. Yet the means by which such education can help remain ill-understood. The onus rests upon those like the contributors to this book to share what they have learned so that teachers new to inter-professional education need not reinvent the wheel.

Conventional wisdom holds that undergraduates need to discover their professional identities and distinctive expertise before being exposed to learning with other professions. But negative stereotypes towards other professions all too easily form during undergraduate education, in which case beginning practitioners emerge ill-disposed and ill-prepared for collaborative practice. 'Remedial education' is then needed to unlearn negative attitudes and bad habits before working together can begin in earnest.

Many universities have introduced shared modules across pathways for students entering different professions to optimise choice and ensure best use of specialist teaching resources. Moves to introduce inter-professional education into the undergraduate curriculum are therefore going with the grain, but experience teaches that sitting side by side in the same lecture theatres does little or nothing to cultivate understanding and mutual respect between professions. That depends upon interactive learning between the parties and upon the application of that learning to collaborative practice. It is here that the five examples of undergraduate inter-professional education in this book promise to be so helpful.

In turn, they demonstrates how:

- learning was built around a model of care to which both nursing and social work students in the field of learning difficulties were invited to subscribe
- innovative learning methods helped midwifery and medical students to understand respective roles and responsibilities
- joint sessions enabled final-year medical students and newly qualified nurses to learn from each other about acute care in an inter-professional skills centre
- ethical issues introduced into joint seminars for medical and nursing students helped them to appreciate different points of view and 'bond'
- placements on an inter-professional training ward developed profession-specific skills whilst also promoting teamwork and insight into the roles of others

All these projects were evaluated, adding to the growing evidence base about the effectiveness of inter-professional education. Weaknesses are reported squarely in the hope that others may avoid the same pitfalls. Plainly, there is more to inter-professional education than compiling core curricula.

Here then is a distinctive contribution to the burgeoning literature on inter-professional education ably reviewed by Stuart Cable to provide a wide-ranging backdrop that musters argument and evidence. It falls to Tony Leiba and Sally Glen, respectively, to set the scene and point up the salient issues.

Reference

Secretary of State for Health (2000) *The NHS Plan*, London: Department of Health. Cm 4818–1

HUGH BARR
Professor Emeritus
School of Integrated Health
University of Westminster
Chairman, UK Centre for Advancement of Inter-Professional Education
(CAIPE)

Preface

In the past, multi-professional education experiences occurred largely by chance in practice settings where the needs of the client, patient or the situation compelled traditionally orientated professionals to work together. With the increased use of multi-professional healthcare teams, many universities and employing agencies have developed programmes for multi-professional groups of students. The multi-professionals' exposure is primarily intended to increase the present and future professionals' ability and willingness to collaborate with one another in the care of users and patients.

The focus of this book is pre-registration, university-based, multi-professional education initiatives. The aim is to bring together current experience and future developments in multi-professional education. It is intended to offer ideas and practical guidance to those developing multi-professional curricula in the changing climate of health and social care

Chapter 1 explores the question, why the current interest in multi-professional education? This chapter suggests that the current emphasis on a greater need for integration and collaboration between professionals is not simply a product of greater professional awareness or more acute sensitivity to the needs of users but rather a product of the interrelationship of developments in policy, education and practice. Each of these factors is considered. The chapter concludes by suggesting that the introduction of multi-professional learning and teaching cannot be considered in isolation. Whilst moves towards integrated programmes for health and social care professionals are undoubtedly in evidence, the explicit objectives are often unclear. There appears often to be a prevailing idea that it is common sense that if students learn together, they will be better prepared to work together. However, the evidence for this viewpoint may be inconclusive and possibly contradictory.

Chapter 2 raises the highly pertinent question, do we need multi-professional education? In answering this question, the observation is made that it is increasingly difficult to meet the needs of individuals in modern society, as fragmented services of specialists and experts struggle with and are seldom successful in solving interrelated problems. However, the professions providing health and social care are in transition, and compounded social changes have rendered their relationships to each other, and to the wider society, increasingly challenging and uneasy. At a glance these circumstances may suggest a combination of situations that will inhibit multi-professional co-operation, but the opposite may be taking place. There is increasing recognition of changing demands and pressures on practitioners and a less narrow and functional view of users. In order to address and illuminate these issues, this chapter examines some perspectives of multi-professional education. The dominant themes are: the defining of terms; some of the circumstances which create opportunities for multi-professional education; multi-professional assumptions; theories of multi-professional education; multi-professional education and the future.

Chapter 3 describes the development, implementation and evaluation of a joint training programme, integrating learning disability nursing and social work into one education and training programme leading to two full professional awards – registration as a learning disability nurse (RNMH) and qualification with a diploma in social work (DipSW). This chapter argues that joint training programmes between health and social care can prepare practitioners for the new, more integrated context in which future health and social services are likely to be delivered. This chapter includes reflections on the challenges encountered and on what has been learned since the programme began.

Chapter 4 describes the planning, implementation and evaluation of a programme of teaching on the topic of normal labour to a group of first-year student midwives and third-year medical students. The aim of the programme is to provide a multi-professional learning environment aimed at not only improving knowledge on the topic of normal labour but also to increase awareness of professional roles. The constraints which present during the planning phase of a multi-professional education programme are identified. These constraints include problems with timetabling, huge discrepancies in numbers of students and the different learning methods in place. Despite these difficulties, the programme proved successful, judging by the evaluations of students and staff. This initiative also produced a shift in attitudes about professional roles and both cohorts of students had more knowledge of the other's responsibilities within a labour ward. Chapter 5 describes a short, inter-professional programme in acute care, involving final-year medical students and newly qualified nurses. This chapter emphasises that it is important to ensure that students following different professional programmes of study 'learn with and from each other' and are not simply in the same room being taught together. The aim of the programme was to improve working relationships through better communication and a better understanding of each other's role. The authors suggest that learning individual clinical skills is probably most efficiently achieved in uni-professional groups. On the other hand, if the group is inter-professional, some learning about each other's professionalism may occur, but there is a danger that students may leave having gained a better understanding of each other's role but unable, for example, to cannulate, or vice versa. As a means of teaching a range of new clinical skills to newly qualified staff nurses and senior medical students, such a course is probably not effective. However, as a means of helping the participants refine and develop existing skills and increase their understanding of the role of another healthcare professional, such a programme appears to have potential.

Chapter 6 describes shared teaching in ethics between pre-registration nurses and undergraduate medical students. During their training the nursing and medical students meet three times for shared sessions in ethics. These sessions take place at the junior, intermediate and senior levels of training. The global aim is to enable the students to develop personal/professional ethical and moral reasoning to enhance patient care. The reason why ethics was chosen as a topic for shared learning and teaching is that, due to advances in medical knowledge and technology, healthcare professionals are required to be more receptive and sensitive to ethical issues. The chapter describes the development, implementation and evaluation of shared learning and teaching in ethics. To achieve progress to date has required vision, determination, courage, considerable goodwill and support from all participants.

Chapter 7 describes, from the evaluator's perspective, the development and pilot phase of an interprofessional training ward placement for medical, nursing, occupational therapy and physiotherapy students. The training ward model was pioneered in Sweden and adapted in the light of the Swedish experience and evaluation, and also to meet the needs and aspiration of service providers, educators and students in inner and east London. The evaluation findings are focused upon seven major themes: real life; learning and teaching; problem-based approach; team duties; preparation for training ward experience; training ward patients and impact of the training ward on service delivery. The authors suggest that this initiative has the potential to develop into a valuable mature project that provides an innovative educational experience for students and staff development opportunities that are unique in the UK.

Chapter 8 concludes the book by identifying four themes which have evolved from Chapters 1 to 6. These themes are: multiple stakeholder perspectives; an integrated approach to care; a system sympathetic to innovation and an evidence-based agenda. Chapter 8 argues that if multi-professional education is to become a reality, innovative new approaches are required. Major reviews will be necessary over the next few years within pre-registration and post-registration programmes to allow for future developments of multi-professional learning opportunities across nursing, midwifery, medicine, dentistry, social work and the professions allied to medicine.

1

The Context – Why the Current Interest?

Stuart Cable

Introduction

One of the overriding challenges of modern healthcare is to create systems which function in a coherent, seamless manner in order to address the complex emotional, social, psychological and pathological problems with which patients present. This challenge has created a need to bring together separate but interdependent health and social care professionals.

Leathard (1994) and Øvretveit *et al.* (1997) propose that changes in healthcare demand a move from the historical position of comparatively discrete professional roles to one which emphasises integration and collaboration. This is not simply a product of greater professional awareness or more acute sensitivity to the needs of patients but also a product of the interrelationship of developments in policy, education and practice.

Each of these factors will therefore be considered in turn. Broad trends that have influenced each in relation to the concept of 'multi-professionalism' will be considered. The definition of the term 'multi-professionalism' is however complicated and terminology highly interchangeable encompassing ideas of 'integration' (Wilson, 1998), 'partnership' (Department of Health, 1997), 'teamwork' (Headrick *et al.* 1998), 'interdisciplinary collaboration' (Mariano, 1989) and 'professional boundary blurring' (Allen, 1997). Definitions will therefore be considered elsewhere (Chapter 2) and the terminology adopted in this chapter will, as appropriate, be determined by that used in the original papers. The text also contains a number of boxes that contain detail of policy documents and research studies through which the reader can reflect on the circumstances in which the move towards multi-professionalism is taking place.

Multi-professionalism in policy

The influence of the World Health Organisation

Leathard (1994), in a wide-reaching review of the emergence of 'interprofessional education and working' recognised that the World Health Organisation (WHO) has had a considerable influence on the development of inter-professional initiatives. In particular she cites the importance of the 'Health for All by the Year 2000' initiative, (World Health Organisation, 1984); however, the idea of 'interdisciplinary integration' within healthcare has been prominent in WHO policy/discussion documents since the early 1970s.

An early paper produced by the World Health Organisation (1973) highlighted deficiencies in the preparation of medical students to work in healthcare teams. The WHO Committee proposed that greater inter-professional integration would increase the recognition of the unique skills of different professions, increase role satisfaction, increase public appreciation of health-care teams and provide more effective, holistic care.

Criticism was made of the implementation of these proposals in achieving their goals (Fulop, 1976). However, failures were suggested to be due to organisational rather than educational influences, namely the separation of training institutions and service delivery units. More recently Tope (1996) gave currency to this criticism describing the existence of 'A wide chasm exist between academic goals, service requirements and consumer expectations in a constantly changing socio-economic climate'. This observation is disconcerting in light of the changes that have taken place in the professional education of nurses and midwives with the transfer from hospital-based colleges of nursing and midwifery to the higher education sector (Glen, 1999). Despite the academisation of the profession and an increased emphasis on the development of theoretical foundations for nursing practice, a recent review of 'fitness for practice' through pre-registration programmes acknowledged the need for closer links between education and service (UKCC, 1999).

Continued discussion of the issue of education and practice documentation prevailed through WHO publications; however, the bodies commitment to holistic patient care and the requirements this created for teamwork and interdisciplinarity were powerfully re-emphasised in the report *Learning Together to Work Together* (World Health Organisation, 1988). However, as with much of the literature on multi-professional education, the commitment was given with a some evidence of the relationship between 'multiprofessional education of health personnel' and its role in 'achieving health for all'.

A British policy response

The structures proposed by the WHO undoubtedly affected the UK health policies. In particular, the three-tier strategy advocating primary, secondary and tertiary care developments (World Health Organisation, 1979) resulted in a trend in policy which moved the delivery of services towards care in the community, for example the *Cumberlege Report* (1986), NHS & Community Care Act 1990 (Department of Health, 1990), *The New NHS Modern, Dependable* (Department of Health, 1997). This placed the onus for much of the service provision on the primary and social care services. In turn, policy placed an emphasis in its directives on primary healthcare teams for example *Care in the Community* (DHSS, 1981), *Primary Health Care: An Agenda for Discussion* (DHSS, 1986). Whilst this closer integration between services had broad support the literature is littered with reports of the breakdown of communications between the different sectors of health and social care organisations, for example the Clyde, Report, 1992 (Figure 1.1). This was despite the early recognition in the WHO report that each sector should 'function in working relationship with the others'. (World Health Organisation, 1979). However, the recognition of the value of integration of health and social services, and an awareness of the complexity of problems which users of the

(D) THE JOINT APPROACH

15.29 While there is a general recognition that in cases of child abuse it is important to follow the course of a 'joint approach' there is some lack of clarity in the understanding of that principle and how it should operate in practice. Even the terms 'co-operation', 'collaboration' and 'co-ordination' are each open to definition, . . . There is a growing understanding that child protection protection is the business of all the agencies not the monopoly of one. It is plainly not sufficient simply to define it in terms of a requirement of all agencies to work with the common end of securing the welfare of the child as if all were united as one agencies. The distinct statutory functions of the principal agencies . . . have to be recognised and respected . . . The essence of the joint approach is a full sharing of the information and intentions of each agency so that the action of one is not prejudiced by any action of the other. It does not imply that all must be involved in every action to be taken by any one but that there is synthesis and harmony in the acting of all of them with a view to creating the greatest benefit and the least disturbance to the child whose interests are paramount.

15.30 One particular practical advantage of the co-operation is the securing that tasks such as medical examination or interviewing, which more than one authority wish to carry out are arranged and carried out jointly, so as to avoid the child being subjected to the unnecessary repetition of such experiences. But the co-operation does not end there. There should be the fullest sharing of information and thinking . . .

15.33 One practical step towards securing a greater degree of practical co-operation is by the organisation of joint training. Another is the preparation of joint guidelines. Each agency should not draw up its own guidelines in isolation. Moreover after inter-agency discussion a common procedural guideline should be prepared with which both agencies will be familiar. Such guidelines would identify the particular actions which will be specific to the responsibility of each agency.

Reflection points

* What local examples of joint working between healthcare or health and social care workers can be provided to demonstrate the Clyde Reports recommendations in action?
* How could joint training be organised between the professions? What are the benefits and potential pitfalls of such an initiative?

Figure 1.1   The Clyde Report: a failure of multi-professional function and recommendations for action

services present, has not necessarily resulted in the development of clear and co-ordinated policy in relation to either global directives or local need. Loxley (1997) illuminates a series of conflicts within the health and social care system which have at least in part been the product of the political philosophies of successive governments. These conflicts whilst not easily resolved, need to be recognised and acknowledged in future policy. The key areas of potential conflict Loxley proposes include arguments in the areas of:

* care versus cure
* central versus local control
* bureaucratic versus collegiate structures
* professional versus managerial dominance
* public versus private funding
* integration versus separation of services, professions and skills.

Policy needs to be designed reflecting the recognition of conflicts present within the system in order that it might promote improved working relationships. An example of a government move to address some of the clinical conflicts by offering guidance on routes to best clinical practice was outlined in the White Paper, *The New NHS Modern, Dependable* (Department of Health, 1997) and the NHS Plan (Department of Health, 2000). This paper outlines plans to set up a new, national, evidence-based performance framework, a commission for health improvements, an institute of clinical effectiveness and further research and development programmes. However, the medical profession remains a dominant power within healthcare (Mackay *et al.*, 1995) and therefore the role of nursing, midwifery and professions allied to medicine in the future of these developments remains to be seen. Mackay *et al.* (1993) have also argued that the trend towards multi-professionalism in policy development might be a covert route to curbing the freedom and autonomy of clinicians. For example, changes in the healthcare management in the 1980s resulted in the loss of nursing's a right to be represented at senior management level. One might also argue that medical professions have been undergoing a period of sustained assault the result of which may be a significant reduction in their clinical freedom and greater control by management (Mackay *et al.*, 1995). Indeed, even within a context of higher education Barnett, 1990 recognised that one of the potential outcomes of interdisciplinarity might be increased control of disciplinary groups by professional managers.

Mackay *et al.* (1995) argue that policy designed to move healthcare towards market values has resulted in a concerted challenge to the dominance of the professions.

> By replacing professional ideas and ideals of performance with those of the government the dominance of professionals has been weakened... Primarily through the initiatives seeking efficiency and effective use of resources, the activities of professionals are now circumscribed.

Mackay *et al.* also propose that the introduction of policy, introduced in the 1980s and 1990s based on market values within the health service, lead to 'a spirit of competition' with emphasis not only on the purchaser–provider split but also involving attacks on the professions. Thus, tensions were created by aiming for co-operation in a context of finite resources, in which hospital and community were encouraged to work together but in which the balance of finance had been tilted from the acute sector to primary care.

The policy document for healthcare, *The New NHS Modern, Dependable* (Department of Health, 1997) which followed a change in government after 18 years of Conservative party rule came with the expectation of a new political philosophy. In the introduction to the document, the Prime Minister, Tony Blair, stated that this new policy marked a turning point for the NHS replacing the 'internal market' with 'integrated care'. The policy proposed teams of local GPs and community nurses working together in primary care groups, which in turn would be required to work with local authorities and NHS trusts. However, financial arrangements for different staff remain inconsistent with nurses generally being salaried staff whilst GPs retain 'independent contractor status'.

Hospital clinicians were also expected to provide a greater contribution to service planning through service agreements with primary care groups. Thus the relationship that recurs throughout the document is based on 'partnership'; partnership between staff, between trusts, primary care groups and local authorities and, most emphasised, partnership with patients. A consultation document recently produced by the Department of Health on future workforce planning (Department of Health, 2000) places considerable emphasis on teamworking across professional and organisational boundaries and flexible working arrangements. Multi-professionalism is therefore firmly on the political agenda. It is to be seen whether education and practice can deliver it.

Multi-professionalism in education

Professional education, higher education and employment

Central to any professional education programme is a concern to prepare skilled practitioners competent to practice in their particular specialist arena (While, 1994). Barr (1996) suggests that the goals of multi-professional education are to develop appropriate attitudes and motivations for working with other professions and the competences to practice collaboratively (Barr, 1998). However, Coit Butler (1978) suggests that no universal agreement exists among educators as to what constitutes competence.

Definitions of professionalism often emphasise the tribal and protectionist nature of the organisations (Beattie, 1995). Friedson (1970) defines the use of the term 'profession' as opposed to 'occupation' which, '...lies in legitimate organised autonomy – that a profession is distinct from other occupations in that it has been given the right to control its own work'. However, as boundaries between professions become blurred one may argue that this distinctiveness may diminish and a subsequent deprofessionalisation or alternative definition of a profession may emerge (Walby *et al.*, 1994). Traditionally, entry to most professionals was under educational control. It required the mastery of certain specialised theoretical knowledge and the application of that knowledge to practice in order to solve problems in the field. Thus, formal training and credentialing has created a sub-culture with specific codes of conduct and ethical practice relationships with patients and other vocations (Jayawickramarajah, 1993).

Millerson (1973) observed a number of changes over time in professional education: greater specialisation and occupational diversity and away from practical education towards a strong theoretical base (as has been seen most markedly in nursing and midwifery education within the last decade); barriers to restrict access to the profession, and restriction of choice at different levels of the educational system. If these factors, designed to restrict and control entry, are taken as elements of the professionalisation process then again the professions may be seen to be under assault from a move to vocational credit schemes which will act 'to dissolve conventional intellectual as well as institutional conventions which limit the mobility of students' (Higher Education Quality Council, 1994).

Whilst education may have traditionally driven practice, one of the more current influences upon professional education, and indeed higher education generally, has been the nature of employment and the demands of the employer. Harvey *et al.* (1997) describe a situation of 'symbiosis between the changing nature of jobs as a result of organisational change and the ability desire and enthusiasm of graduates to "grow" jobs'. They describe a situation in which employers want adaptable people who can rapidly fit into a workplace culture, function in teams, exhibit strong interpersonal and communication skills and aid in the transformation of organisations.

Hurst (1999) suggests, for example, that the shape of future healthcare employment and delivery might require a new model of education based on the delivery of a multi-skilled workforce. The educational framework proposed for this change is multi-disciplinary in nature and based on a modular structure comprising six different elements (HSMU, 1996):

1. common core modules for all health care professionals
2. medical and scientific modules for some
3. generic care modules for the majority of students
4. therapists modules for the majority of students
5. additional education modules for generic carers or therapist working in such areas as ICU (intensive care unit)
6. continuing education modules for all health carers.

This educational framework which would bring the different professions closer together for their learning demonstrates a number of similarities to developments occurring in Sweden in the early 1980s (Areskog, 1995). The organisational and curricular structure was designed 'to create flexibility and adaptiveness to future social changes in occupational roles, MPE a multi-professional research are intended to develop new thinking, new roles and competencies, new responsibilities and areas of interest within healthcare and its delivery.'

This move to closer integration of professional education underlies a general trend in higher education. Bernstein (1971) describes the outcome of a movement towards a less compartmentalised form of educational design in terms of an 'integrated curriculum'. This type of curriculum involves the creation of opportunity for active connections to be made between different subject matter in the 'interests of relevance' to practice (Beattie, 1995). However, Bernstein recognised the dynamic nature of education describing a cyclical process through two extremes, the 'integrated curriculum', in which things are put together, and a 'collection curriculum' which has been more traditional in medical and nursing education, in which subject matter was kept apart. For example, Atkinson (1981), in an ethnographic exploration of a medical school, identified how its organisation and processes were designed to maintain the segmentation of knowledge into areas distinct to the ideology of medicine. Similarly, in an analysis of nurse education in Scotland, Melia (1987) identified what she describes as 'compartmentalization' and 'segmentation' as key features of the system.

Johnston (1978) proposes that the situation of integration is seen as threatening to those firmly located within the collection curriculum ethos 'because impure, weakly classified learning with a variety of options and combinations offers the threat of transgressing familiar social and moral boundaries' (Beattie, 1995). However, Beattie proposes that this current turn in favour of integrated curricula, delivered for example through integrated modular programmes or problem-based learning approaches, may provide a powerful opportunity for 'transcending the tribalism of health professionals'.

Barnett (1990) argues for the promotion of this trend towards integration which he views as a vital to the cognitive development of students, who can respond flexibly to the needs of society. He argues that the prolonged emphasis on disciplinary purity has been detrimental: 'academic disciplines are a major impediment to the realization of a liberal conception of higher education. A liberal conception cannot be sustained amidst barriers to student's intellectual inclinations'. Barnett proposes a number of aims or motivations that justify the pursuit of 'interdisciplinarity' (Table 1). This table outlines the plurality of perceived benefits of

Table 1.1   Aims of inter-disciplinarity

Aim/Motivation	Rationale
Educational	Broadening dimension through integration of elements; developing relationships between learning and actual 'life' situations
Epistemological	Contrasts conceptual frameworks, truth criteria, levels of objectivity, methodologies, creating context for new kinds of thinking
Communicative	Development of common discourse across disciplinary cultures
Pedagogical	Encouragement of co-operation among educational staff of different disciplines and exposure of students to wider range of teaching strategies
Preparation for labour market	Greater capacity for adaptability, flexibility and improved development of personal transferable skills
Technocratic	Development of courses grounded around particular functional spheres/ roles

Managerial	Multi-disciplinarity redistributes power relationship in favour of management, therefore flexibility and possibly cost savings can be introduced into subject delivery
Informatory	Breakdown of discrete academic communities that have resulted in a failure to communicate with the wider public
Normative	Provision of education as a vehicle which puts knowledge into service for a political end, e.g., political or social reform
Rational	Unification of reasoning around a particular theme to create a supra-rationality of, e.g., health
Critical	Development of capacity to challenge central suppositions of and interest structures of particular disciplines

Source: Barnett (1990, pp. 178–83)

closer integration in learning among the professions. For example, it may address claims of over-exclusivity of subject matter, which has denied access to a wider audience and sustained a protectionist attitude among the professions; it may also transfer power from the clinical professions to professional managers. However, partition of knowledge has been acknowledged as the traditional form in healthcare education. Cribb and Bignold (1995) illuminate this partition in their analysis of the research culture prevailing in medical schools. When contrasted with the emerging nursing research culture it emphasises the fundamental challenges to multi-professionalism. Whilst nursing has embraced more holistic approaches to care and reflective and interpretive paradigms, medicine, and arguably professions allied to medicine, largely continue to reside in the positivist paradigm.[1] Medicine the culture of medicine remains firmly embedded in professional-scientific discourse nursing has adopted a more holistic, reflective knowledge base. Thus, unless fundamental differences in the paradigmatic stances of different professional groups can be achieved, this would appear to be a significant impediment to closer working relationships as different professions may be founded within conflicting paradigms. In medicine the emphasis on facts and empiricism will conflict with a nursing culture founded on reflection and interpretation. If so, the ground for common discourse may be scant.

Multi-professional educational delivery in health care

Szasz (1969), an early advocate of integrated education for the health professions, expressed his concern about the separatist and competitive culture that arose from academically and often geographically distinct healthcare education programmes. He argued that traditional education methods encouraged and reinforced individual achievements at the expense of collaboration and co-operation. Mason and Parascondola (1972) argued for the redesign of the whole educational structure. They argued that students should start to work together at the commencement of their careers. The initial stages of the educational preparation taking place through a core curriculum based on the following assumptions; students learn to function as team members and sharing learning will support this. The mode of working will be economically more efficient, and inter-professional learning will contribute to increased inter-professional collaboration.

Indeed the converse view was put forward by Mazur *et al.* (1979) who argued that students should not be integrated in the early stages of their educational development but rather should develop a role identity of their own which they can then contextualise within the wider multi-professional arena.

Howard and Byl (1971) undertook a three-year study of integrated educational programmes including students of medicine and other health care professions. They found that whilst satisfaction with the educational process of all other groups went up, those of medical students went down.

An extensive study of attitude change among teachers, social workers and community workers at the Moray Institute in Edinburgh (McMichael *et al.*, 1984) highlighted a more positive perception by teachers of social workers and community workers. However, this was not reciprocated. Similarly, Carpenter (1995) undertook one of the few pre-test, post-test evaluation studies of attitude change in medical, nursing and social work students following a one-week integrated course of study and found a generally positive trend, but this was by no means universal. There is also a paucity of data to support the implicit notion that inter-professional education will have a long-term impact on practice.

Studies also suggest that whilst outcome measures may provide some benefit in evaluating educational interventions, there is also much emphasis to be placed on educational process, including consideration of joint planning, participant commitment and clarity of objectives (Davidson and Lucas, 1995). Loxley (1997), for example, suggests that collaboration is based on the presence of 'charismatic enthusiasts' whilst Friedson (1970) proclaims that organisational and environmental influences are more likely to have an impact on behaviour than professional preparation.

Harden (1998) has called for more explicit focus on the most appropriate modes of educational delivery. He proposes utilising a three-dimensional model which makes explicit the relationship between particular learning contexts, curriculum goals and multi-professional education strategies. This approach would appear to be useful in focusing on the efficacy of particular strategies. For example, Parsell *et al.* (1998) identify that 'Placing small classes of nursing, dental and therapy students with much larger classes' of medical students to be taught anatomy and physiology is no longer an acceptable example of effective shared teaching'. Indeed, evidence exists that such a form of 'shared teaching' may reinforce stereotypes and harbour resentment (Areskog, 1988) (Figure 1.2). However, Tope (1996), in a feasibility study, *Integrated interdisciplinary learning between the health and social care professions*, Collating data from 1500 students, argues that learning about inter-professional working is best achieved when students interact in 'real-life' situations, that is in the direct provision of patient care. Freeth and Nicol (1998) share this position and describe a study in which they attempt to simulate practice. Mixed groups of newly qualified staff nurses and fifth-year medical students were brought together in a clinical context to work through patient scenarios. However this study, whilst described as a 'success', also highlights a common problem, that of delivering resource-intensive learning methods to large numbers of students.

A review of a range of studies therefore highlights that evidence is mixed on the most appropriate and feasible curriculum designs

Carpenter and Hewstone (1996), in a pre-post test study of attitude change amongst medical, nursing and social work students based the rationale for the education initiative on the contact hypothesis, a framework upon which negotiations in complex, conflict situations have been based and which place significant emphasis on creating contacts between respective parties. The factors underlying success in this domain include:

- institutional support
- equal status of participants
- positive expectations
- co-operative atmosphere
- successful joint-working
- concern for and understanding of the differences as well as similarities
- experience of working together as equals and perception that members of the group are typical and not just exceptions to the stereotype.

Considerable planning of multi-professional educational encounters are therefore evidently required to prepare the respective parties and such factors as location, stage, content, duration and frequency, assessment and learning/teaching styles must be considered (Barr, 1996).

Reflection points

- How can the circumstances upon which successful multi-professional contacts are hypothesised to occur be created? What might be the process of preparation for such encounters?
- What are students concerns about learning with other students and what learning strategies might be most appropriate for addressing these?

Figure 1.2   Creating contact between students: a rationale for multi-professional education

or modes of delivery for effective multi-professional education. The plurality of required outcomes, for example by managers, clinicians, patients, students and educators, is perhaps unlikely to allow simple linear relationships to be defined between educational input and practice outcomes. The discussions outlined here have exemplified a complex web incorporating educational process, organisational design, professional and personal differences. However, unless there is some notion of success as educationalists and researchers begin to evaluate the meaning, contexts and processes of multi-professional teaching and learning then there is a danger of multi-professional education 'becoming another untested article of faith' (Loxley, 1997) that may serve no one.

Despite considerable efforts in the educational arena a recent systematic review identifies that there is no rigorous quantitative evidence to substantiate the effects of inter-professional education (Zwarenstein *et al.*, 1999). Whilst this chapter does not conclude that there is no value in such moves the research base on which to found future educational direction appears to be limited. Whilst this may be so, Miller *et al.* (1999: 222) recognise that education alone should not be the sole strategy for developing more integrated practices:

> In the acute sector, organisational policies have driven working practices towards greater patient throughput by filling as many beds as possible, and staff turnover is high. Despite good intentions, [...], the development of highly collaborative working practices may be practically impossible. [...] It is a mistake to think that education alone can achieve better collaborative practices.

The practice context will therefore be reviewed.

Multi-professionalism in practice

The ascendancy of the healthcare 'team'

West (1996) argues that the concept of teams and teamworking in delivery of services and products has become the dominant philosophy within many organisational settings. He provides evidence to support this trend, citing studies which demonstrate that this can result in increased effectiveness in both quality and quantity of services (for example Guzzo and Shea, 1992; Weldon and Weingart, 1993). However, in a historical overview of healthcare teams Brown (1982) argues that, whilst the need for teams is well recognised, talk of teams has been dominant in healthcare for at least thirty years. Banta and Fox (1972) argued that the reality of healthcare teams was largely 'high-sounding rhetoric' because participants were too diverse and unfamiliar with each other to function as such; nurses reacted to physicians in a traditionally deferential way and physicians took charge of the teams. More recent studies suggest this situation to be still largely the case (West and Slater, 1996).

Numerous educational and policy changes have occurred in the last 25 years since Banta and Fox's (1972) paper. However, Headrick *et al.* (1998) also recognise a major flaw in the context for creation of team cultures: 'the reality of practice is often that the professionals with whom one must collaborate are the people who happen to be there.' The result of the prevailing organisational climate is a frequently reported failure of healthcare teams to set aside time for regular meetings to define objectives and clarify roles, apportion tasks, encourage participation and manage change (Field and West, 1995).

The reality of the situation is therefore that whilst, healthcare professionals speak of teams, they tend to work autonomously due to differences of professional routine, fears of loss of identity and differences in education and training. Indeed, the differences between the professions are often so great that Mackay (1993) is driven to comment: 'their worlds are so dissimilar that it is surprising that so much common ground has been established in day to day working relationships.'

At a structural level the differences that mitigate against multi-professional teams are also striking. Dingwall and McIntoch (1978), for example, argued that without according equal status, power and prestige inter-professional collaboration is futile, but evidence of significant differentials prevail as the Audit Commission (1992) reported: 'Separate lines of control, different payment systems... all play a part in limiting the potential of multi-professional, multi-agency teamwork... for those working under such circumstances efficient teamwork remains elusive'.

Relationships in healthcare

The relationships between health professionals, in particular those of doctors and nurses, have been much studied in the literature (Stein *et al.*, 1990; Mackay, 1993; Allen, 1997; Wicks, 1998) (Figure 1.3). Stein *et al.* (1990) describe a much-cited, complex 'game' which retains the dominance of the doctor whilst enabling the nurse covertly to participate in decision making. Svensson (1996) argues, however, that the relationship between doctors and nurses is rather the product of continuous negotiation between them, a social structure based on 'a negotiated order'. Allen (1997) builds on this perspective by considering the changing boundaries between medical and nursing work, as nurses move into areas of medical work that were traditionally the sole domain of doctors. This, she argues, is likely to create an increased need for inter-occupational negotiation due to associated tensions as staff and patients redefine the different roles. However, her clinical observations, although limited in scope, reveal little evidence of the tensions one might

Walby *et al.* (1994) undertook a study of medical and nursing staff working in a range of hospital settings to identify causes of conflict. They found that the causes of breakdown in relations were frequently workload and staffing levels but also differences in routine and priorities. Key areas of conflict resulted from:

- low staffing cover
- stress and tiredness
- theatre lists running over time
- bed availability, e.g. admission, discharge and outliers
- communication failure, e.g. bleeps
- variability in routines, e.g. ward rounds, handovers
- consultant absenteeism/disinterest
- different medical/nursing budgets.

The study undertaken in both teaching and district general hospitals gives an example of a surgical department which stood out in terms of teamworking from all others to a degree that could not be explained by levels of funding. Important factors identified by staff to explain this finding included competence of consultants and ward sisters, stability of nursing workforce, small size of department and few consultants, good inter-consultant relations, approachability of consultants and also supportive inter- and intra-professional networks.

Reflection points

- What issues do students identify from their clinical experiences which facilitate/inhibit multi-professional working practices?
- Which factors could staff/students address to improve working relationships and minimise conflict and how might they go about putting such strategies in place?

Figure 1.3   Hospital practice: the causes of conflict in the medical and nursing teams

expect from change. Allen argues that it appears that social mechanisms are in place which largely retain the order of health-care delivery and nurses participate in medical decision making to a degree that belies their position in the formal organisational hierarchy. However, this observation provokes a question of 'what is considered as the practice of "multiprofessionalism"'?. Is it a reconstitution of roles, and relationships or the sustenance of the traditional, hierarchical order in which the doctor retains dominance? Indeed, an argument may be made that it may be organisationally most appropriate within the present system in which legal accountability is carried by the doctor (Mackay *et al.*, 1995) to retain a long-established, hierarchical relationship between the professions.

Wicks (1998) argues that there is a need to question the current divisions of labour in healthcare which she claims are based on 'a nineteenth century conception of master/servant gender appropriateness'. Whilst she acknowledges that these relationships may be masked beneath a social context in which respect and politeness smooth inequitable relationships, she suggests that the result of these divisions is that the medical problem dominates all other aspects of the patients life.

The dominant position of the medical profession has perhaps become so much the norm that one may ask how it could be different. Beattie (1995) however proposes alternative models of healthcare delivery which, encouraged by the growth in inter-professional health studies, might bring about a realignment of the boundaries of healthcare work:

- *The biotechnological model of health* focuses on 'mechanical defects' in individuals and sets out to rectify these in light of biomedical sciences and technology.
- *The biographical model of health* focuses on troublesome life events that are personally significant for the individual, and aims to help the person develop strategies for coping with these.
- *The ecological model of health* concerns the risks and hazards of human environments and seeks social intervention to reduce risks and protect the vulnerable.
- *The communitarian model of health* in which social groups and social movements mobilise to share their health concerns and which engage in co-operative advocacy and campaigning for change.

These models, Beattie (1995) argues, cut across traditional tribal boundaries and create opportunities for a different division of labour, ones in which the common ground between professions becomes more significant than traditional differences.

Hurst (1999) highlights a more functional model of health practice that might at least blur the boundaries between professions if not address the tensions, a model based on 'multi-skilling'. This model proposes that health carers should be not be restricted by function, traditional compartmentalisation or overspecialisation (HSMU, 1996) but rather should be equipped to provide the services required by the patient. Whilst this move might serve the purpose of personalising patient care by reducing the need for patients to interact with fewer staff, it fails to address how staff from different professions would respond to each other within this new structure. Additionally, some evidence exists to support the need for practitioner specialisation, for example in accident and emergency services (Audit Commission, 1996). Nevertheless, this move could have important ramifications for professional educational development.

Conclusion

The introduction of multi-professional teaching and learning cannot be considered in isolation. Moves towards integrated programmes for health professionals are undoubtedly in evidence and at various stages of development. There appears often to be a prevailing idea that it is common sense that if students learn together they will be better prepared to work together.

The trend may in party be due to financial and political expediency on the part of educational administrators needing to be seen to be doing something in the face of government and service demands. Policy and practice rhetoric both appear to support a general trend towards multi-professionalism but the route to its achievement is less clear. This is in part due to the fact that there are numerous interpretations of what a successful outcome in respect of closer collaboration between health and social care professionals actually means.

Even where agreement exists on the definition of multi-professionalism in practice the educational competencies which would support organisational processes remain unclear. West (1999) advocates the promotion of 'reflexivity' in preparing practitioners. Health and social care professions' texts abound with the concept of reflective practice. One might therefore question whether uniprofessional work in this domain will result in multiprofessional outcomes without the need for specific shared learning experiences.

Considering the challenges of multi-professional teaching and learning, the logistics of bringing students together, the curriculum changes required, the efforts of staff and students to be expanded and the upheaval of health and social care institutions to facilitate contact, it is essential that the move is evidence based and ultimately will serve the recipients of the service, namely the patients.

Note

1   An argument might be made that primary health care medicine is a notable exception to this contention.

References

Allen, D (1997) The nursing–medical boundary: a negotiated order?, *Sociology for Health and Illness*, **19**, 498–520.

Areskog, N (1988) Editorial: The need for multi-professional health education in undergraduate studies, *Medical Education*, **22**, 251–2.

Areskog, N-H (1995) Multi-professional education at the undergraduate level. In Soothill, L, Mackay, L and Webb, C (eds), *Interprofessional relations in health care*, pp. 125–39, London: Edward Arnold.

Atkinson, P (1981) *The Clinical Experience. The Construction and Reconstruction of Medical Reality*. Farnborough: Gower.

Audit Commission (1992) *Homeward Bound: A new course for community health*. London: HMSO.

Audit Commission (1996) *By Accident or Design. Improving Services in England and Wales*. London: HMSO.

Banta, D and Fox, R (1972) Role strains of a health care in a poverty community, *Social Science and Medicine*, **6**, 607–722.

Barnett, R (1990) *The Idea of Higher Education*. Buckingham: Open University Press.

Barr, H (1996) Ends and means in inter-professional education: towards a typology, *Education for Health*, **9**, 341–52.

Barr, H (1998) Competent to collaborate: towards a competency-based model for interprofessional education, *Journal of Interprofessional Care*, **12**(2).

Beattie, A (1995) War and peace among the health tribes. In Soothill, K, Mackay, L and Webb, C (eds), *Interprofessional Relations in Health Care*, 11–26, London: Edward Arnold.

Bernstein, B (1971) *Class, Codes and Controls, Volume 1*. London: Routledge.

Brown, T M (1982) An historical view of healthcare teams. In Agich, G J (ed) *Responsibility in Health Care*, Dordrecht, Holland: Reidel Publishing Company.

Carpenter, J (1995) Interprofessional education for medical and nursing students: evaluation of a programme, *Medical Education*, **29**, 265–72.

Carpenter, J and Hewstone, M (1996) Shared learning for doctors and social workers: evaluation of a programme, *British Journal of Social Work*, **26**, 239–57.

Clyde Report (1992) *Report of the Inquiry into the Removal of Children from Orkney in February 1991*, Edinburgh: HMSO.

Coit Butler, F (1978) The concept of competence, *Educational Technology*, **18**, 7–16.

Cribb, A and Bignold, S (1999) Towards the reflexive medical school: the hidden curriculum and medical education research, *Studies in Higher Education*, **24**(2), 195–209.

Cumberlege Report (1986) *Neighbourhood Nursing: A Focus for Care*. Report of the Community Nursing Review, London: HMSO.

Davidson, L and Lucas, J (1995) Multi-professional education in the undergraduate health professions curriculum: observations from Adelaide, Linkoping and Salford, *Journal of Interprofessional Care*, **9**, 163–76.

Department of Health (1990) *NHS and Community Care Act*. London: HMSO.

Department of Health (1997) *The New NHS Modern Dependable*. London: HMSO.

Department of Health (2000) *The NHS Plan*. London: HMSO.

DHSS (1981) *Care in the Community*. London: DHSS.

DHSS (1986) *Primary Health Care: An Agenda for Discussion*. London: HMSO.

Dingwall, R and McIntosh, J (1978) Teamwork in theory and practice. In Dingwall, R and McIntosh, J (eds), *Readings in the Sociology of Nursing*. Edinburgh: Churchill Livingstone.

Field, R and West, M (1995) Teamwork in primary health care 2: perspectives from practices, *Journal of Interprofessional Care*, **9**, 123–30.

Freeth, D and Nicol, M (1998) Learning clinical skills: an interprofessional approach, *Nurse Education Today*, **18**, 455–61.

5555555

Friedson, E (1970) *Profession of Medicine. A Study of the Sociology of Applied Knowledge*. New York: Harper and Row.

Fulop, T (1976) New approaches to a permanent problem, *WHO Chronicle*, **30**, 433–41.

Glen, S (1999) The demise of the apprenticeship model. In Nicol, M and Glen, S (eds), *Clinical Skills in Nursing. The Return to the Practical Room?*, Basingstoke: Macmillan – now Palgrave.

Guzzo, R and Shea G (1992) Group performance and intergroup relations in organisations. In Dunette, M and Hough, L (eds), *Handbook of Organisational Psychology 3*, 269–313, Palo Alto: Consulting Psychologists Press.

Harden, R (1998) AMEE guide No.12: Multi-professional education: Part 1 – effective multi-professional education: a three-dimensional perspective, *Medical Teacher*, **20**, 402–8.

Harvey, L, Moon, S, Geall, V and Bower, R (1997) *Graduates' work: organisational change and student attributes*, Birmingham: Centre for Research into Quality, University of Central England in Birmingham.

Headrick, L, Wilcock, P and Batalden, P (1998) Interprofessional working and continuing medical education, *British Medical Journal*, **316**, 771–4.

Higher Education Quality Council (1994) *Choosing to change. Extending access, choice and mobility in higher education*, London: Higher Education Quality Council.

Howard, J and Byl, N (1971) Pitfalls in interdisciplinary teaching. *Journal of Medical Education*, **46**(9), 772–81.

HSMU (Health Services Management Unit) (1996) *The Future Healthcare Workforce*. Manchester: HSMU.

Hurst, K (1999) Educational implications of multiskilled health carers. *Medical Teacher*, **21**, 170–3.

Jayawickramarajah, P (1993) The Effectiveness of Problem-Based Curriculum in Medical Education. In *Faculty of Educational Studies*, **450**, Southampton: University of Southampton.

Johnston, K (1978) Dangerous knowledge: a case study in the social control of knowledge, *Australian and New Zealand Journal of Sociology*, **14**, 104–12.

Leathard, A (1994) Interprofessional developments in Britain: an overview. In Leathard, A. (ed.), *Going Inter-Professional. Working Together for Health and Welfare*, 3–37. London: Routledge.

Loxley, A (1997) *Collaboration in Health and Welfare. Working with Difference*. London: Jessica Kingsley Publishers.

Mackay, L (1993) *Conflicts in Care: Medicine and Nursing*. London: Chapman and Hall.

Mackay, L, Soothill, K and Webb, C (1995) Troubled times: the context for inter-professional collaboration. In Soothill, K, Mackay, L and Webb, C (eds), *Interprofessional Relations in Health Care*, 5–10, London: Edward Arnold.

Mariano, C (1989) The case for interdisciplinary collaboration. *Nursing Outlook*, **37**, 285–8.

Mason, E J and Parascondola, J (1972) Preparing tomorrow's health care team, *Nursing Outlook*, **20**(11), 728–31.

Mazur, H, Beeston, J and Yerxa, E (1979) Clinical interdisciplinary health team care: an educational experiment, *Journal of Medical Education*, **54**, 703–13.

McMichael, P, Irvine, R and Gilloran, A (1984) *Pathways to the professions: research report.* Edinburgh: Moray House College.

Melia, K (1987) *Learning and Working. The Occupational Socialization of Nurses.* London: Tavistock Publications.

Miller, C, Ross, N and Freeman, M (1999) *Shared Learning and Clinical Teamwork: new directions in education for multiprofessional practice*, London: English National Board for Nursing, Midwifery and Health Visiting.

Millerson, G (1973) *Education in the Professions*, Cook, T (ed.). Methuen.

Øvretveit, P, Mathias, P and Thompson, T (1997) *Interprofessional working for health and social care.* Community Health Care Series. Basingstoke: Macmillan – now Palgrave.

Parsell, G, Spalding, R and Bligh, J (1998) Shared goals, shared learning: evaluation of a multi-professional course for undergraduate students, *Medical Education*, **32**, 304–11.

Stein, L, Watts, D and Howell, T (1990) The doctor-nurse game revisited, *Nursing Outlook*, **38**, 264–8.

Svensson, R (1996) The interplay between doctors and nurses – a negotiated order perspective, *Sociology of Health and Illness*, **18**, 379–98.

Szasz, G (1969) Interprofessional education in the health sciences, *Millbank Memorial Fund Quarterly*, **47**, 449–75.

Tope, R (1996) *Integrated interdisciplinary learning between health and social care professions. A feasibility study.* Aldershot: Avebury.

UKCC (1999) *Fitness for Practice.* London: UKCC.

Walby, S, Greenwell, J, Mackay, L and Soothill, K (1994) *Medicine and nursing. Professions in a changing health service.* London: Sage.

Weldon, E and Weingart, L (1993) Group goals and group performance, *British Journal of Psychology*, **32**, 307–34.

West, M (1996) *Handbook of Workgroup Psychology.* Chichester: Wiley.

West, M (1999) Communicating and teamworking in healthcare, *NT Research*, **4**, 8–17.

West, M and Slater, J (1996) Teamworking in primary health care: a review of its effectiveness, London: Health Education Authority.

While, A (1994) Competence versus performance: which is more important? *Journal of Advanced Nursing*, **20**, 525–31.

Wicks, D (1998) *Nurses and Doctors at Work. Rethinking Professional Boundaries*. Buckingham: Open University Press.

Wilson, J (1998) Integrated Care Management, *British Journal of Nursing*, **7**, 201–2.

World Health Organisation (1973) Continuing education for physicians, Technical Report Series NO. 534, Geneva: WHO.

World Health Organisation (1979) Primary health care in Europe, Euro Report No. 14, Geneva: WHO.

World Health Organisation (1984) Health for All 2000, Copenhagen: WHO Regional Office.

World Health Organisation, Steering Group on Multi-professional Education (1988) Learning together to work together for health. The team approach. Geneva: WHO.

Zwarenstein, M, Atkins, J, Barr, H, Hammick, M, Koppel, I, Reeves, S (1999) A systematic review of interprofessional education, *Journal of Interprofessional Care*, **13**(4), 417–24.

2

Multi-professional Education: Definitions and Perspectives

Tony Leiba

Do we need multi-professional education? In answering this question one might make the observation that it is increasingly difficult to meet the needs of individuals in modern society, as fragmented services of specialists and experts struggle and are seldom successful in solving interrelated problems. For example, a child with medical problems not only needs healthcare but may also need help from social carers and educationalists.

The professions providing health and social care are in transition. Compounded social changes have rendered their relationships to each other and to the wider society increasingly challenging and uneasy. Most of these professions have varying degrees of image problems, and external pressures have induced some soul searching and responses to criticisms. These pressures have shown up divisions, boundary conflicts and inter-professional rivalries.

However, at a glance these circumstances may suggest a combination of situations that will inhibit multi-professional co-operation, but the opposite may be taking place. Most of these professions operate from a common environment, shared interests are growing, and the underlying processes and dynamics of issues relevant to health and social care are not unique to individual professions. There is increasing recognition of changing demands and pressures on practitioners and a less narrow and less functional view of users.

In order to address and illuminate the aforementioned issues, this chapter will examine some perspectives of multi-professional education. The dominant themes will be: the defining of terms; some of the circumstances which create opportunities for multi-professional education; multi-professional assumptions; theories of multi-professional education; multi-professional education and the future.

Defining terms

The World Health Organisation (1988) considers 'multi-professional' to be concerned with health-related occupations with different educational backgrounds learning together during certain periods of their education, with interaction as the process which will facilitate future collaboration. The World Health Organisation's definition needs to be broadened so that other groups, such as social workers, the police and teachers, can become a part of multi-professional initiatives. These professionals need to communicate and interact effectively with health professionals, as was seen in the Butler-Sloss Report on Child Abuse in Cleveland (Butler-Sloss, 1988).

Pirrie *et al.* (1998) offers a description of multi-professional education as a generic term for a range of teaching and learning situations where students from different health and social care professions come together to enhance their understanding of elements in their professional practice, thereby equiping the professionals to provide a service which is intended to be seamless. Generally the term multi-professional education implies teaching and learning opportunities involving more than one profession. Over the years shared learning, multi-professional learning and inter-professional learning have all been used. What everyone is really discussing is how to facilitate health and social care professions and professionals to learn and work together.

In inter-professional education all the students learn together. They may learn in role-playing situations so as to learn together and so promote collaborative practice. These learning activities provide for greater interactivity between the different professional participants, resulting in people learning with, from and about each other. A distinction between inter-professional and multi-professional education is made by Parsell and Bligh (1998) who argue that 'inter-professional' is used to describe learning activities involving two professional groups and 'multi-professional education', to describe learning activities involving three or more professional groups.

Multi-professional education might be hindered by the tension between research and practice, which has powerful institutional support. The argument is that the research base differences between the professions does not help in developing integrated learning. Another argument is that entry gates are not compatible and so programme organisers are faced with the problem of finding the correct level to pitch classroom activities. In some instances it is possible that a professional group might dominate and so reinforce stereotypes. Professional identity, standards and value systems might be perceived as conflicting with multi-professional education. Associated with this is the role of professional bodies in maintaining distinctive professional cultures. For example, the requirements of professional bodies in terms of number of hours of theory and clinical practice makes logistic problems for curriculum planners.

A common question which is constantly being asked is at what stage is multi-professional education perceived to have most impact, and in what areas of the curriculum is it likely to be most successful? Pirrie *et al.* (1998) identify less interest in multi-professional education at pre-registration levels. This may be because there is a need for each profession to develop first their own identity. However, Horder (1996) has emphasised the value in starting multi-professional education in the early stages of training to anticipate the development of negative stereotypes. There are, however, strong arguments supporting the model whereby each profession first studies independently, acquiring the mastery of its own profession prior to multi-profession learning. Pre-registration courses between different professions have taken place at Salford University, Sheffield Hallam University and Suffolk College. At the post-registration stage there are more courses and multi-professional initiatives, but medical graduates are more attracted to recognised medical courses which are funded through their postgraduate allowances and vocational training.

Here multi-professional education will mean, as argued by Barr (1996), the teaching of common content to a mixed group of health and social care professionals, with such a teaching and learning enterprise occurring at both pre- and post-registered levels and aimed at promoting collaborative practice in the delivery of health and social care. There are, however, concerns from the professions and the professionals, who envisage threats in standards of care and that the evidence in support of multi-professional education being insufficiently robust.

Opportunities for multi-professional education

Health and social care documents concerned with service developments, educational priorities, the development of a seamless service and the promotion of continuity of care through more effective professional co-ordination have been available from the Department of Health, the National Health Service Executive and the Social Services Directorate since the early 1970s (Leathard 1994, 1997). The Barclay Report (1982) stated that collaboration between social workers and other services should be on a basis of mutual respect, and that arrangements for collaboration must be planned so that factors which may affect relationships are understood, so preventing tension by both managers and practitioners.

The paper *Working for Patients, Education and Training* (Department of Health 1989a) resulted in the transfer of nursing, midwifery, the professions allied to medicine, physiotherapy, occupational therapy and radiography into universities, with new opportunities for multi-professional education. The paper also specified the separation of purchasers and providers and the need for purchasers to ensure that opportunities for multi-professional education were developed.

The Department of Health (1989b) White Paper, *Caring for People in the Community: Community care in the next Decade and beyond* defines collaboration as a partnership of joint working between authorities and agencies involved in planning and delivering services to the community. In its discussions of the principles of assesment it states that some users will suffer from several problems or disabilities and so need both health and social care. Therefore the assessment process must be able to embrace flexibility and must be as broad a view as possible.

Calman (1994) in his paper 'Working Together: teamwork', argues that the aims of a team do not occur spontaneously but have to be discussed debated and agreed jointly.

The Department of Health (1996a, 1996b) document clearly states that evidence-based practice for clinical effectiveness in primary care must be linked to the need to develop professional knowledge through the provision of more opportunities for multi-disciplinary learning and continuous education. The White Paper on the future of the NHS, (Department of Health 1997) makes collaborative care and partnerships a central issue. Pittilo and Ross (1998) argue that professionals, whether they are primary practitioners or teachers, will continue to experience considerable changes and continuing re-evaluation of traditional roles unencumbered by historical and professional boundaries, and that such a situation has implications for multi-professional education. A consultation document by J.M. Consulting (1998) for the Department of Health has raised the question of multi-professional or uni-professional regulation for nurses, doctors and the professions allied to medicine. The support for this joint regulation is that they increasingly work together and that the regulatory framework could be more user driven rather than profession driven.

There is a need to address generic and profession-specific knowledge and skills which are necessary for multi-professional education and work. To date there is only limited research. Therefore there is a need for more funding to be available to research this area. Furthermore, the pressure to reduce costs in education and training must be balanced with the need for academic staff to keep up to date through research and clinical practice.

Multi-professional assumptions

Essentially multi-professional education involves several levels of understanding: an awareness of the existence and the nature of multi-professional education and a acceptance of its legitimacy; a thorough understanding of one's own profession so that one can be clear about what it can contribute to solve a problem and what other professions can contribute; and finally, the confidence to develop and maintain multi-professional contacts and the facility to overcome professional barriers.

Societal complexities and the advance of technological specialisation means that a number of people will have problems
that can no longer be solved by one profession. If the professions
embrace these complexities and changes, they must be aware that
where professional interests overlap a decision must be made as
to who and which profession will be responsible for what. Another
challenging area is cross-professional disagreements, for example
ethical issues around confidentially. Some professionals are highly
sensitive to the confidential nature of user information. Such issues
must be resolved in specific cases if full co-operation and fewer
professional disagreements are to be achieved. Working with the
mentally ill and the disabled also requires differences between
the professions and the individual professional to be resolved if
co-operation and effective working together is to become a reality.

Multi-professional education must also address sexism and
racism. Leiba (1994) suggested that differences between the professions around the issues of sex/gender and race/ethnicity can
contribute to difficulties in arriving at common goals at the site
of the delivery of health and social care services. In the case of
sex/gender issues, Hearn (1982) argued that the patriarchal work
environment results in the replication of relationships in which
the power of men over women is sustained, resulting in perceived
conflicts between the professions being in part a power struggle
between men and women. Therefore, if multi-professional education and practice where women and men are individual participants is being considered, an awareness of sex/gender issues
around power relations and oppression at work must be addressed
(Hugman, 1991).

Turning to race and ethnicity, a multi-professional approach
requires each profession to examine its ideologies and practices
vis-à-vis anti-discriminatory, anti-racist and anti-oppressive delivery
of health and social care. Discrimination against people on grounds
of sex, religion, sexual orientation, race/ethnicity and disability is
prevalent in society generally, and in health and social care pro-
visions and delivery in particular. Professionals must therefore
realise that as part of a society which maintains such discrimination they must examine their own bias and deal with it. For
example, Baxter (1992) provides information and analysis on
the effects of discrimination in providing care for ethnic groups
with learning disabilities, while Day (1994) provides insights into

the pervasive forms of discrimination and racism in systems and institutions.

User direction, client participation, carer involvement and patient power are words used to denote that consumerism in health and social care are here to stay. People expect to be fully informed about treatments, care and services, and to have a greater say in decisions previously made by the professional. The effect of user participation on multi-professional education and practice might be addressed through the relationship between the professional and the person by the words the professional uses to describe the people they serve (Steinberg, 1992; Biggs, 1993; Meyer, 1993). For example, some social workers call the people they serve 'clients' or 'service users'. These words suggest a different relationship from 'patient', which doctors and nurses call the people they serve patients (Ovretveit, 1997).

The words used in interactions between the professional and the public form the basis on which the relationship between the person and the professional is constructed, and they also assume certain behaviours and attitudes. If the users' position and power is less passive and more participatory, does this situation affect the way professionals work together? Does it make multi-professional practice more or less difficult? Ovretveit (1997) argues that, in planning multi-professional education, curriculum developers must attend to the insights of the sociology of the professions, which has built up a knowledge about how professions relate and the power struggles between them (Hugman, 1991).

Some professionals may view an active, questioning and challenging person as difficult to help. Such professionals might wince at the use of the words 'consumer' or 'customer', which suggest the opposite of patient, giving the person more power in dealings with the professional. Further, some professionals might feel that these words emphasise the commercial and economic value of the person rather than humanity. Whilst 'user' discourages dependency, it can give the impression of exploitation rather than partnership. If the professionals are working multi-professionally, can they agree on a term which is right for a particular service? If not, why not?

Multi-professional and inter-professional working might also be affected when practitioners seek to be more open with users about their condition or problem. Generally users now seek more information about their assessment, diagnosis and prognosis and are not prepared to be fobbed off. Looking at doctors and nurses, it has been traditionally difficult for the nurse to know how much, or what, to tell. In the past the doctor made it clear what the nurse could say. However, as nursing and other health and social care professionals move towards increasing autonomy and user advocacy, conflict may arise between them, for example, when the user is given the assessment and prognosis details and these differ from the doctor's, or differ from each professional information (Steinberg, 1992). There is therefore a need for closer rather than less multi-professional co-operation, to be open to users means that the professionals have to be more open with each other. In order to work multi-professionally the professionals must problem solve and agree policies about disclosure to patients.

Another area where user – practitioner relationships may affect multi-professional working is the right to access of users to their case records (*Access to Personal Files Act 1987*, *Access to Medical Report Act 1988*, *Access to Health Reports Act 1990*). The concern here is whether one profession allows access to a record which holds information about the user given by other professionals. Again, a useful way of working multi-professionally is for professionals to discuss and agree a common policy about access and disclosure.

Theories of multi-professional education

According to Pirrie *et al.* (1998), evidence exist which supports the benefits of multi-professional education at pre-registration and post-registration levels in Europe, the United States of America and the World Health Organisation (Areskog, 1988, 1992, 1994; Goble, 1994; Casto, 1994; Clarke, 1993 and WHO, 1988). Their evaluations, however, show mainly the impact of multi-professional education on attitudes rather than on improved care to users.

Spencer (1987) has suggested that multi-professional education has evolved in part in response to the increasing complexities of contemporary societies. More and more traditional professions are finding that their competencies are outstripped by the challenges people bring to them. These challenges are interwoven and they require not only a common framework of knowledge but also an understanding which respects differences in the response to the multiplicity of users' needs. Professionals therefore need to be educated about the role, values, ideologies, culture and beliefs of the different professions. Underpinning such an educational perspective must be tolerance and respect between the professions and the professionals.

Frederick (1995) has suggested that there are within Western civilisation debates about unity and multiplicity, arguing that there is a tendency both towards greater differentiation in organisations and towards co-operation and integration. Perhaps the development of highly differentiated professions and the equal call for multi-professionalism and integration reflects this preoccupation. Similarly, Schon (1992) suggested that professions in America were becoming aware of zones of practice, situations of complexity and uncertainty, which require artistry to successfully complete their tasks. He also reminded us to be aware of the multiplicity within a profession that is likely to be competing with schools of thought within that profession, and that professions change, split, reorganise, merge and generally respond to changes in their environment.

Szasz (1969: 152) offers a short but useful definition of 'multi-professional' as 'preparation of student for collaborative service relationships'. Such a multi-professional education might be achieved through shared learning by the placing of various professional disciplines in the same classroom; through intra-professional learning, where different specialists groups share the same course and classroom; by inter-professional learning, where various professional disciplines participate in a course or courses dealing with inter-professional issues such as language, ideology, values, ethics and discrimination; and through joint learning, where students complete a course which leads to two or more professional qualifications.

Harden (1998) has offered a three-dimensional model of multi-professional education. The three dimensions are: the context in which the multi-professional education is to be applied (this includes the phase or stage of education, the category of students and the teaching methods to be employed); the curriculum goals and the expected outcomes of the programmes; the approach to the multi-professional education being adopted, which includes Harden's (1998) 11 steps continuum between discipline or subject-based teaching at one end and multi-professional at the other. This continuum is a move from received learning to learning through interaction between different professionals. Also it is a move from theoretical learning to experience-related learning of the real work world of the professionals. This three-dimensional model of multi-professional education offers a tool and insights into possible planning, implementation and evaluation.

Multi-professional education and the future

Multi-professional education is difficult to provide, implement and maintain because of educational health and social care professionals takes place in separate institutions. They are funded differently, and they all have professional cultures which have different emphasis on operations and administration. Goble (1994) argues that many professionals think that precious time should not be spent on multi-professional activities. It is also difficult for educators who have only experienced the uni-professional model to understand and to teach the knowledge and skills in a multi-professional curricular.

Interests and developments in multi-professional learning in Europe began in the 1970s. In Sweden, at the University of Linkoping, multi-professional developments were initiated in 1986 whereby courses were run for laboratory technologists, nurses, occupational therapists, physicians, physiotherapists, and supervisors of social services and community care. All started the first year with a common ten-week multi-professional course. After this introductory study the different curricula for the different professional groups contained multi-professional sessions throughout the programme, which ended with a three-week team training course. Student and tutor evaluations provided evidence that the experience was on the whole positive (Areskog and Lundh, 1987).

In the United Kingdom, at Exeter University, the first multi-professional continuing education scheme for the professions allied to medicine and doctors in general practice was organised by the Postgraduate Medical School. This started in 1975 as a series of evening lecturers and later as day-release courses with successful students gaining an MSc. degree (Goble, 1994). South Bank University started an MSc in Interprofessional Health and Welfare Studies in 1990 (Leathard, 1992). The Marylebone Centre trust and the University of Westminster have developed post-graduate courses. A further development in the UK has been the Centre for the Advancement of Interprofessional Education in Primary Care and Community Care (CAIPE). The aim of CAIPE is to promote development, practice and research into interprofessional education for practitioners and managers involved in primary health and community care (Goble, 1994).

In France the University of Bobigny, Paris Nord, introduced a unique course in 1984 concerned with orienting students towards different health professions – nursing, dentistry, medicine midwifery, psychology, biology and health service management (d'Ivernois, 1987).

The University of Limburg, Maastricht, in the Netherlands has developed a course where all the health sciences students have the same programme in the first year. In the remaining years the student concentrates on the chosen programme for half the time. The rest of the time is devoted to a joint programme in health sciences and general science (Goble, 1994).

In Linkoping, Sweden in 1987 the European Network for Development of Multi-professional Education in Health Sciences (EMPE) was formed. The aim of the network was to promote the concept of multi-professional education in health sciences through the facilitation and exchange of information, personnel and experiences. The development of joint research and evaluation was identified as a priority along with active support for educational institutions facilitating multi-professional research.

Inter-professional and multi-professional initiatives in the United States of America is in as similar stage of development as in Europe. However, much of their work started as early as 1948 with the Cherasky team homecare concept at Montefore Hospital (Cherasky, 1949). This history of teamworking, which provided the impetus for later multi-professional education and working, is partly derived from the model of team healthcare delivery developed by the Peckham Experiment at London's Pioneer Health Centre in the 1990s (Baldwin, 1982). Now universities across the United States of America provide multi-professional courses. At the same time the Ohio Interprofessional Commission, which started out to provide collaborative education across a number of human disciplines, is developing nationwide. The commission is a collaboration between academics and practitioners to provide pre-service courses and continuing education experiences to prepare professionals for inter-professional practice. The professions involved are from education, law, dentistry, medicine, nursing, public administration, social work and theology (Casto, 1994).

Within the context of evidence and practice multi-professional education is not easily identifiable as a good. What are the benefits? Does it result in better care for users? These are questions for which we have little researched evidence. Since this is a new field, researchable problems are in abundance and considerable work needs to be done of a theoretical nature. The assumptions upon which multi-professional education and practice are based are mostly untested. Substantial work must be done on the effects of multi-professional education on practice itself. Some questions for research could be: do professionals who take multi-professional courses actually practice multi-professionally?; what is the impact on users of multi-professional services? Such questions require complex research approaches because they are value laden and saturated with untested assumptions.

Providing multi-professional education requires extraordinary organisation and managerial skill, and it cannot become a reality without institutional and inter-institutional commitment. The complexity of issues within multi-professionalism makes it a suitable candidate to become a specialist area for research and expertise. Advanced degrees will proliferate as research evidence grows and graduates assume leadership and managerial positions in organisations.

Our circumstances within the wider society, in our families, individual lives, professions and institutions are not likely to become less complex, since health and social care matters have many facets, and no one professional, however well prepared and with the best of intentions, can address all the relevant aspects. Therefore our challenge is to collaborate across all the professions and so give a positive multi-professional service to users.

References

Access to Health Reports Act 1990. London: HMSO.
Access to Medical Reports Act 1988. London: HMSO.
Access to Personal Files Act 1987. London: HMSO.

Areskog, N (1988) The need for multi-professional health education in undergraduate studies, *Medical Education*, **22**, 251–2.

Areskog, N and Lundh, L (1987) The Health University of Linkoping, Sweden, *EMPE* newsletter **1**, 1–3.

Areskog, N (1992) The New Medical Education at the Faculty of Health Sciences, Linkouping University – a challenge for both students and teachers, *Scandinavian Journal of Social Medicine*, **2**, 1–4.

Areskog, N (1994) Multiprofessional education at the undergraduate level. In Soothill, K, Mackay, L and Webb, C (eds), *Interprofessional Relations in Health Care*. London: Edward Arnold.

Baldwin, D C (1982) The British are coming: some observations on health care teams in Great Britain. In Pisaneschi, J (ed.), *Interdisciplinary Health Team Care: Proceedings of the Fourth Annual Conference*, Lexington, Kentucky: Centre for Interdisciplinary Education, University of Kentucky.

Barclay Report (1982) *Social Workers: Their Roles and Tasks*, London: Bedford Square Press.

Barr, H (1996) Ends and Means in Interprofessional Education: Towards a Typology, *Education for Health*, **9**, 341–52.

Baxter, C (1992) Providing care in a multi-racial society. In Thompson, T and Mathias, P (eds), *Standards in Mental Handicap: Keys to competence*. London: Bailliere Tindall.

Biggs, S (1993) User participation and interprofessional collaboration in community care, *Journal of Interprofessional Care*, **7**(2), 151–60.

Butler-Sloss, E (1988) *Report of the Inquiry into Child Abuse in Cleveland, 1987, Cm413*, London: HMSO.

Calman, K (1994) Working Together: teamwork, *Journal of Interprofessional Care*, **8**(1), 95–9.

Casto, M (1994) Interprofessional work in the USA: education and practice. In Leathard, A (ed.), *Going Interprofessional, Working Together for Health and Welfare*. London: Routledge.

Cherasky, M (1949) The Montefore Hospital home care programme, *American Journal of Public Health*, **39**, 29–30.

Clarke, P G (1993) A typology of multidisciplinary education in gerontology and geriatrics: are we really doing what we say we are?, *Journal of Interprofessional Care*, **7**(3), 217–27.

Department of Health (1989a) *Working for Patients, Education and Training*. Working Paper 10. London: HMSO.

Department of Health (1989b) *Caring for People in the Community: Community Care in the next Decade and Beyond. Cm849*. London: HMSO.

Department of Health (1996a) *Primary Care Delivering the Future*. London: HMSO.

Department of Health (1996b) *The National Health Service with Ambitions*. London: HMSO.

Department of Health (1997) *The new NHS*. NHS White Paper, London: HMSO.

Day, M (1994) Racial Discrimination: Professional Implications, *Journal of Interprofessional Care*, **8**(2), 135–40.

d'Ivernois, J F (1987) The Faculty of Medicine of Bobigny University Paris Nord, *EMPE* newsletter, **1**, 1–3.

Frederick, C (1995) A holographic approach to holism, *Journal of Interprofessional Care*, **9**(1), 9–15.

Goble, R (1994) Multi-professional education in Europe. In Leathard, A (ed.), *Going Interprofessional: Working Together for Health and Welfare*. London: Routledge.

Harden, R M (1998) AMEE guide No. 12: Multi-professional education: part 1 – effective multi-professional education: a three-dimensional perspective, *Medical Teacher*, **20**(5), 402–8.

Hearn, J (1982) Notes on patriarchy, professionalism and the semi-professions. *Sociology*, **16**(2), 184–202.

Horder, J (1996) The Centre of the Advancement of Interprofessional Education, *Education for Health*, **9**(3), 397–400.

Hugman, R (1991) *Power in the Caring Professions*. London: Macmillan Press, now Palgrave.

J M Consulting (1998) *Review of Nurses, Midwives and Health Visitors Act 1997*. consulting document, Bristol: J M Consulting Ltd.

Leathard, A (1992) Interprofessional developments at South Bank Polytechnic, *Journal of Interprofessional Care*, **6**(1), 17–23.

Leathard, A (1994) *Going Interprofessional: Working Together for Health and Welfare*. London: Routledge.

Leathard, A (1997) Interprofessional Education and the Medical Profession: The Changing Context in Britain, *Education for Health*, **10**, 359–70.

Leiba, T (1994) Interprofessional approaches to mental health. In Leathard, A (ed.), *Going Interprofessional: Working Together for Health and Welfare*. London: Routledge.

Meyer, J (1993) Participation in care: A challenge for multi-disciplinary teamwork, *Journal of Interprofessional Care*, **7**(1), 57–66.

Ovretveit, J (1997) How patient power and client participation affects relations between professions. In Mathias, P and Thompson, T (ed.), *Interprofessional working for health and social care*, London: Macmillan – now Palgrave.

Parsell, G and Bligh, J (1998) Interprofessional Learning, *Post-graduate Medical Journal*, **74**, 89–95.

Pirrie, A, Wilson, V, Harden, R M and Elsegood, J (1998) AMEE Guide No. 12: Multiprofessional education: Part 2 – promoting cohesive practice in health care, *Medical Teacher*, **20**(5), 409–16.

Pittilo, R M and Ross, F M (1998) Policies for Interprofessional Education: Current trends in the UK, *Education for Health*, **11**, 285–95.

Schon, D A (1992) The crisis of professional knowledge and the pursuit of an epistemology of practice, *Journal of Interprofessional Care*, **6**(1), 48–65.

Spencer, M H (1987) Impact of Interprofessional Education on Subsequent Practice, *Theory and Practice*, **26**(2), 134–40.

Steinberg, D (1992) Informed consent: Consultation as a basis for collaboration between disciplines and between professionals and their patients, *Journal of Interprofesional Care*, **6**(1), 57–66.

Szasz, G (1969) Interprofessional Education in the Health Sciences, *Milbank Memorial Fund Quarterly*, **47**, 449–75.

World Health Organisation (1988) *Learning together to work together for health*. Geneva: WHO.

3

Joint Training for Integrated Care

Dave Sims

Introduction

It is recognised that the starting point for the design of professional education and training should be the skills required for practice. Although this is apparently self-evident, it is only relatively recently that competency-based approaches have been espoused as the means by which to ensure these skills are developed. This chapter discusses the integration of two professional training programmes and their respective competencies to develop a new 'joint practitioner' in learning disability nursing and social work. The emerging practitioners have been shown to:

- possess enhanced skills in inter-professional working and collaboration
- have a breadth of knowledge and networks which can be employed in their work with people with learning disabilities
- bring an extra dimension to their work when employed in either nursing or social work
- be aware of different professional cultures and perspectives and be able to work across professional boundaries

The value of an integrated and holistic approach combining health and social care approaches is not a new concept in professional practice (see Chapter 1), but in the field of learning disabilities it has found an important resonance given that the vast majority of people with learning disabilities now live in the community and not in hospital. The commitment to strive for this approach has led, in the last ten years, to the important development of 'joint training' in the field of learning disabilities. Joint training programmes completely integrate learning disability nursing and social work into one education and training programme leading to two full professional awards – registration as a learning disability nurse and qualification as a social worker.

There are currently six such programmes in England, and by the year 2001 over 300 joint practitioners will have qualified from them. The programmes generally take three years to complete and are founded on the premise of a high degree of role overlap between these two professions.

Two recent, parallel developments in social policy have underlined the relevance of this integrated approach to professional education and training. *The New NHS* White Paper (1997) sets out how the internal market will be replaced by a system of 'integrated care, based on partnership' (1.3). It promises to ensure this through a new statutory duty for NHS trusts to work in partnership with other NHS organisations, such that co-operation will replace competition (2.24). Primary care groups will include GPs, community nurses and representation from social services, who will work together to establish and abide by the local health improvement programme. One of the stated functions of the groups is to 'better integrate primary and community health services and work more closely with social services on both planning and delivery' (5.9).

This theme of partnership and integration is equally reflected in the *Modernising Social Services* White Paper (DoH, 1998), which promises that obstacles to collaboration between health and social services will be removed to enable pooled budgets, lead commissioning and integrated provision. Reference is made to bringing down the 'Berlin Wall' that can divide health and social services. The aim is to achieve 'flexible partnership working which moves away from sterile conflicts over boundaries' (6.3).

This chapter will explore the development of a programme which, it will be argued, can prepare practitioners for this new, more integrated context in which future health and social services are likely to be delivered. The rationale, underpinning principles, structure and delivery of joint training will be discussed, with particular reference to the programme run at South Bank University. The chapter will include reflection on the challenges encountered and on what has been learned in the nine years since the programme began. Finally, evaluation of this model of training will be considered, with particular reference to a research project undertaken at the university with former students and their employers.

Historical context

One of the major contributory factors leading to the development of joint training in learning disabilities has been the reconfiguration of services since the 1971 White Paper *Better Services for the Mentally Handicapped*. This policy initiative led to the large-scale closure of hospital provision for people with learning disabilities which has taken place over the last 25 years. The move away from hospital provision impacted on thinking around which practitioner should lead in supporting people in the community.

Critiques of hospitals and institutional living had identified poor living conditions, isolation and a philosophy of 'containment' as key problems impacting on care. The question of whether there was a need for nurses in the care of people with learning disabilities came under the spotlight. 'Apart from epilepsy, the amount of serious physical or mental illness amongst them appears to be small', stated Pauline Morris in *Put Away*, published in 1969 (cited in Malin, 1995: 61). If the nursing needs of patients were not judged to be significant enough to justify hospital provision were they enough to justify a separate branch of nursing?

The ensuing debate about 'which practitioner was needed' seemed to be concluded in 1972 when the Briggs Report (DHSS, 1972) proposed a realignment in care for the mentally handicapped between health and social services, and recommended 'A new caring profession for the mentally handicapped should emerge gradually. In the meantime, in the training of nurses in the field of mental handicap, increased emphasis should be placed on the social aspects of care' (Recommendation 74). This controversial recommendation was later reviewed in the *Jay Report* in

1979, which opted for giving the responsibility for training staff to work with people with learning disabilities to CCETSW. The new caring professional would be trained in an equivalent to the CSS (Certificate in Social Service) qualification, a social work training mainly taken up by seconded employees of social services departments. The future for specialised nursing at this point did not look hopeful, until a new government in 1979 decided to reject this plan.

The Jay Report did, however, establish the principle that people with learning disabilities needed to receive support in the communities where they lived in order to help them develop as individuals. Throughout the 1980s multi-disciplinary community mental handicap teams were established which reflected this principle, many of them comprising of both learning disability nurses and social workers.

Joint working between the General Nursing Council and CCETSW then developed over a number of years, looking at ways of introducing common elements into nurse and social work training. As a result of this, two pilot joint training courses were established in the south of England in 1988, leading participants to qualification as both a learning disability nurse (RNMH) and a social worker (CSS).

Local demand for joint training

Whilst hospital closure has clearly influenced the education and training debate at a strategic level, it has also led to local demand from services for new and innovative approaches to training. The South Bank programme arose directly from such local demand. Managers at both the district health authority and other key learning disability services did not believe that either 'pure' social work or nurse training would best equip practitioners in the new community-based services which had been established following the closure of a large long-stay hospital. As one manager subsequently put it when asked why his organisation had supported the programme: 'Social workers do not have the health skills of nurses. There are also elements of social work training that are stronger than nursing, e.g. anti-discriminatory and reflective practice.'

Managers also believed that jointly trained practitioners could become agents of change in services. At a time of large-scale hospital closure, it has subsequently been observed that service managers were often seeking alternative solutions to employing workers with clearly identifiable health or social care backgrounds, in order to avoid the problems thrown up by strong attachment to previous working experiences (Means and Smith, 1994). Joint training appeared to offer one challenge to rigid professional identification or working practices.

The rationale for joint training

As well as the historical development of services, there are three other key aspects of the rationale for joint training in learning disability nursing and social work. The first of these is the undeniable link between social factors and health. Recent policy guidance to NHS learning disability services explicitly recognises the link and calls for a holistic approach, involving:

> close co-operation with local authority colleagues to develop a full range of suitable services that address both health and social care needs. Often it is impossible to separate such needs because people have both. Everyone has health needs if only for health education, promotion and screening. Good social care supports a healthy lifestyle. Therefore health services must view people as a whole and work closely with everyone involved. (NHSE, 1998: i)

The future requirement to undertake joint working is clear, and whether this is co-operation, collaboration or partnership it is arguable that professionals need to be trained to do it. One of the greatest obstacles to be overcome is perhaps the very singular nature of professional training. The fact that many practitioners are trained exclusively in one environment (either health or social, but rarely both) can lead to misperceptions about other environments, cultures and professional values. These misperceptions can lead to barriers to communication, understanding and joint working. Joint training courses train practitioners in both environments, and emerging practitioners have recognised the value of this in developing their understanding of different professional perspectives.

The second aspect of the rationale for joint training returns us to the training and education debate. A comparison of the learning outcomes for learning disability nursing and social work programmes reveals very substantial similarity between the two. Integrating the outcomes together has not proved difficult for programmes to achieve. The role overlap is very significant, although there remain important differences, and this means the two disciplines complement one another when combined into a single programme. Clearly, one of these differences is the health perspective, an aspect of learning disability nursing which has received important re-emphasis in the last few years, coinciding with research evidence that the health needs of people with learning disabilities have not been fully addressed (Mencap, 1997).

The third aspect to the rationale for joint training is the positive impact of that training on integrated approaches to practice. The very processes involved in the training reflect the tensions practitioners often have to grapple with when they embark on joint working. Placements in contrasting settings require students to negotiate and agree learning outcomes and necessitate a flexible but focused 'learning needs led' approach. The fact that practice learning is needs-led makes the process a model for future working, as summed up by the ENB and CCETSW:

> Successful shared learning and joint education and training provide a model for effective collaborative working and an integrated approach to practice. This helps to ensure that the care provided is focused on meeting the needs of those using services. (ENB/CCETSW, 1995)

The structure of the programme

The programme has an intake of 18 students each year. It follows the structure of a three-year Project 2000 nurse training course, being divided into two equal periods of 18 months each, the first being a common foundation programme (CFP) and the second a branch programme where the focus is on work with people with learning disabilities. The normal two-year period of social work training is therefore extended to three and this enables some flexibility around teaching and learning for social work. During the CFP the students undertake 100 days of practice learning in a range of health settings (mental health, maternity, work with children, adult nursing and learning disabilities), before progressing to two long-term placements of 60 days in year two and 120 days in year three. These in-depth placements meet the CCETSW requirements for more extended periods of practice with qualified practice teachers.

In terms of the taught programme, much of the foundation curriculum is common to both social work and nursing, particularly the social sciences. The key difference is that these topics are, in this programme, more likely to be delivered from a nursing perspective, and the joint training students will be sharing their learning with those planning to take up careers in child, adult and mental health nursing. In the branch part of the programme the social work and learning disability aspects are developed much further with the joint training students, in a discreet, smaller group.

Although this kind of integrated curriculum has its critics (particularly those who believe that professional training is about professional *socialisation*), it has been positively evaluated by former students for giving them insight into the range of services and service cultures that reflect the experience of people with learning disabilities. Clearly an integrated training programme such as this does not aim to socialise students into one professional culture more than the other, but to prepare them for both.

Another concern that has been expressed about joint training is that it could lead to a 'generic' worker, with the loss of specialist expertise. The evidence points to quite the opposite conclusion. As far as social work training is concerned, joint training courses intensify the specialism and are proving popular with those with a real commitment to this field of work and with previous experience. Of the only nine social work courses in England offering a pathway in learning disabilities, five are now joint programmes. The importance of nursing in maintaining the learning disabilities specialism must be acknowledged, with a current estimated 1400 students undertaking learning disability nurse training.

A framework of common competencies

A programme that awards two professional qualifications in different disciplines has the obvious challenge of ensuring it meets the outcome requirements of each. Given the similarities in these outcomes, the first step was to develop a framework of competencies that would integrate these outcomes. It was judged appropriate to adopt a competency-based approach from the outset to ensure that assessment of practice was evidence based. This also reflected the CCETSW revision of the Diploma in Social Work in 1995 to a competency-based award. The programme's original competency framework, devised in 1992, was not a complete integration of outcomes, and the year 2 main placement was actually only assessed against social work outcomes for the first two student intakes. This was in part due to the fact that it was originally felt that there were two nursing competencies which could not be integrated within the social work curriculum, these being health promotion and teaching and learning. But by 1996, when the framework was revised, it was clear that there were strong connections between these and social work outcomes, as had been indicated through students' experience in practice placements.

The 1996 Common Competency Framework was developed in consultation with practitioners and practice agencies involved with the programme. There was a balance of representation from learning disability nursing and social work. Two consultation workshops were held to cross reference the UKCC Rule 18a Outcomes for Nursing and the CCETSW six Core Competencies (see Figure 3.1). The first question addressed by the working groups was: what skills, knowledge and values are needed to best support people with learning disabilities? From the answers gathered to this question, the groups went on to link these to the professional requirements for the two trainings, and the course team was then able to draft a framework of eight common competencies for final ratification (see Figure 3.2). This was also informed by the ENB Creating Lifelong Learners indicative curriculum for learning disability nursing (ENB, 1994). The fact that this framework was the outcome of collaboration has undoubtedly given it added value as an assessment tool, being as it was designed with current fitness for purpose in mind.

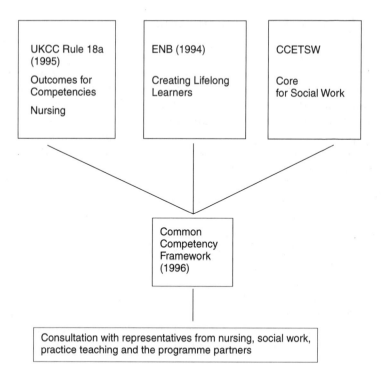

Figure 3.1   The integration of learning outcomes into one common competency framework

Inter-professional competence

One of the benefits of the new Common Competency Framework was that it was fully integrative of nursing and social work and would be used on both main branch placements. As previously mentioned, the earlier framework had only partially assessed students against nursing outcomes in the first main placement. The new framework was also more focused, with the number of assessment criteria having been reduced from approximately 80 to 50. This reduction may have reflected a confidence derived from knowledge that the ENB and CCETSW were working on guidance for joint validation procedures in order to limit the kind of 'complex negotiations with professional and academic

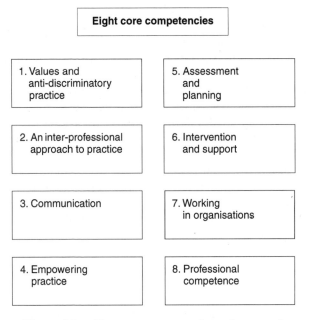

Figure 3.2   The common competency framework

bodies' which joint courses often entail (Bartholemew *et al.*, 1996).

Another improvement was that competency in inter-professional work was made especially explicit, with the inclusion of a competency entitled 'An Inter-professional Approach to Practice'. This requires students to:

- identify both the social and health implications of learning difficulties
- demonstrate the contribution of both nursing and social work skills and knowledge in promoting health and well-being
- integrate health and social care needs in assessment
- demonstrate an understanding of professional roles and manage difference and conflict
- promote inter-agency work and work across professional boundaries, liaising with, co-ordinating and accessing services
- work effectively in a multi-disciplinary setting.

It was important to be explicit about what a jointly trained professional should be able to demonstrate in terms of collaborative working. It is easy to take the above skills for granted or to attribute them to personality characteristics, that is, 'some people are just good at them and some aren't'. Whereas traits such as openness and flexibility may facilitate inter-professional activity, there is undeniably a set of skills that can be learned and perspectives that can be developed. Barr (1998) argues that some of these should be standards of practice for all professionals in the care sector.

Joint practice should result from the application of this competency. This is an orientation towards practice which is holistic, collaborative, flexible in role and based on an anti-discriminatory approach, which incorporates advocacy for health within a social model of disability (Barr, 1998, p. 183).

A programme based on partnership

One of the most tangible benefits of a joint training programme is the potential diversity of support for it from practice. In purely practical terms, a programme such as this can appeal to two different professional networks, nursing and social work. There has, however, been great interest from the voluntary sector whose work with people with learning disabilities often crosses into both of these networks and is increasingly expanding in scope.

CCETSW's requirement of a programme management committee, with committed agency partners overseeing the programme jointly with the education provider, makes for a very constructive foundation for an inter-professional course. The principle of partnership runs through all the processes in which the programme is engaged. It facilitates consultation and involvement at all levels, from strategic decision making and quality assurance to practitioner involvement in recruitment and interviewing, teaching and practice teaching.

The other key area of partnership is the presence of a practice assessment panel to oversee the quality of practice learning and assessment on the programme. The panel comprises five practice assessors from learning disability nursing and social work (one of whom is jointly trained), whose role it is to moderate the assessment decisions of practice teachers on the two main branch practice placements, through the reading of the substantial practice portfolios compiled by student and practice teacher. Being inter-professional in its make up, the panel directly reflects the jointness of the programme and is a means by which the ability of students to integrate their practice, and the ability of the programme to facilitate this, can be monitored and developed.

The panel is particularly involved in assessing the quality of practice teaching on placement, and it was feedback from the panel which prompted the programme to apply for development funding to set up an inter-professional practice teaching course, which is now successfully running. Here nurses and social workers study for the same academic award and, where nurses are practice teaching a student from the joint programme, they are able to be assessed for the CCETSW practice teaching award as well. Participants on the course have clearly developed their own inter-professional awareness and this has been translated into some very successful placements.

Challenges encountered

One of the questions students have sometimes struggled to answer, especially early on in the programme, is whether they are a social worker or a nurse. The issue of professional identity is inevitably of importance on a programme which is challenging it. The support of 'belonging' to either one group or the other, and therefore the certainty of knowing who you are and what your predetermined role is, to some extent eludes the joint practitioner. Students sometimes feel they have difficulty in giving constructive replies to such a question or to the suggestion that they are not a 'real' social worker or nurse.

The programme organises workshops in which some of these issues can be explored. How you answer such questions can be important to self-esteem and confidence, especially when you have deliberately chosen to be involved in a programme which is bringing together two professional perspectives. In these workshops students have thought about how their training is related to improving services and creating a more holistic approach to the needs of people with learning disabilities; how the training reflects recent policy initiatives; and how it gives them a breadth of skills and a good understanding of the different professional contexts experienced by people with learning disabilities.

In addition to helping students to reflect upon their identity and to ensure they are able to evaluate professional boundaries and develop the potential of their joint practitioner role, the programme intentionally places great emphasis on values. This is because it is essential that students have clearly reflected on the relative (power) positions of people with learning disabilities and professional practitioners to ensure that their future practice is sensitive to this and empowering in its effect. Students are encouraged over the three years to critique the negative aspects of some professional behaviour and look to developing an approach which is based on listening to and supporting people first, rather than on 'role-based' assumptions.

For staff delivering a joint programme there are also professional tensions. Compromise is needed in respect of practice experiences, for example. Confidence needs to be invested in professionals of one background to develop learning opportunities for the achievement of some areas of competence they may not have previously addressed or assessed. Currently there are very few jointly trained practice teachers or lecturing staff, so joint training is largely being delivered by those who are singly trained, a fact that is not always lost to the students! What is called for is that staff and practice teachers demonstrate and model the selfsame inter-professional competence that is required of the students. This involves keeping in sight the overall vision and objectives of the programme and working with others of different disciplines to achieve them. It also means offering support to practice teachers in terms of additional visits to placement and offering workshops to address particular training issues.

One of the areas that has often been discussed in relation to the programme is that of the 'balance' between nursing and social work, particularly in respect of practice learning. What *is* an appropriate balance in respect of a joint programme? And how to achieve it? Balance can be discussed from different perspectives: balance between learning disability nursing and social work with people with learning disabilities; between statutory and non-statutory placements; between residential and fieldwork; between purchasing and provision; between placements with people with complex needs and those with people with moderate learning disabilities. There are no easy answers, and there are other factors which can impact on what can be done including, most importantly, the availability of appropriately skilled practice teachers of both disciplines prepared to offer placements.

The programme has adopted a number of approaches to address balance in practice learning. These include: giving students contrasting experiences in their second- and third-year placements; requiring all students to have carried out specific work with a person with complex needs; and ensuring that placement contracts address 'balance' from the outset, such that individual strategies can be established to guarantee work with different practitioners as is required. The two long, in-depth placements can facilitate this individualised approach, and experience has shown that where practice teachers are themselves on the interprofessional practice teaching course, the quality of practice learning experience is markedly high and these issues appropriately negotiated.

The conclusion from several years experience of practice learning in joint training is that the process of placement organisation, is, like many other aspects of joint training, one that requires the engagement of committed individuals to seek the best, most inter-professional learning experiences possible. These experiences are not generally far from reach, though imagination and co-operation may be required to access them. They may also demand of the student the kind of flexibility he or she is expected to demonstrate in practice as a joint practitioner. Thus placement arrangements can themselves be a model for interprofessional work. A student may, for example, spend time in two or even three different environments during his or her final placement, with supervision from practitioners of different disciplines. In their final practice portfolio students are expected to demonstrate how they have integrated their learning from these sources in respect of both health and social perspectives.

Programme evaluation

The movement towards joint training in learning disability nursing and social work has been gradual but sustained, with a great deal of interest being shown in the current programmes by other universities interested in setting up courses. Whilst there is very little research to evaluate outcomes, many practitioners believe this form of training to be particularly useful to supporting people with learning disabilities. This belief appears to emerge from an undeniable logic that a practitioner so trained will be able to unite two important dimensions of people's experience – the health and the social.

Joint training may also be attractive for another reason. It seems to offer a constructive alternative to what has been referred to as the 'medical model'. Although most learning disability services have rejected this model, it is arguably still associated with service provision in some areas, particularly where people still live in hospitals. Perhaps joint training is seen as advantageous because the joint practitioner owes allegiance to a set of values which is derived in part from one profession (social work) which has less connection with medical practice. Joint training incorporates the vital health perspective but within a new framework of a *social* model.

Lessons learned from the previous programmes

Evaluation of the first two 1988 pilot programmes revealed some issues that had an impact on the design of the South Bank programme. One of these was the need for programmes to be integrated and not be modifications of existing programmes. One of the 1988 pilots involved students having their nursing teaching in a different college to their social work teaching. This led to criticism about the disjointedness of the programme. The South Bank programme was deliberately incorporated into a three-year nursing degree structure from the outset, which meant that the social work staff were part of an inter-professional team, albeit numerically much larger in terms of nursing staff. This has generally worked well, and the joint training students have often been regarded as good people to have in the lecture room, as they were sometimes older, outspoken and more willing to give their views during discussions. For the course team, organisation of the programme has been easier, although there have sometimes been tensions in ensuring the specific requirements of CCETSW are met. For example, particular policies have had to be devised which are mandatory for the joint programme (for example policy for the early termination of placements) but at the discretion of the other nursing programmes.

Another issue that arose from the early evaluations of the pilot courses was the difficulty in finding appropriate placements and being able to support practice teachers. The South Bank programme addressed this from the beginning by appointing a practice teaching development worker to organise placements and develop support for practice teaching. This has proved very successful, as it is primarily through this post holder that the partnership with agencies is made a reality. High quality placements can only be secured by carefully building up a network of supporters of joint training over a sustained period of time, by maintaining that network and by adding committed individuals and agencies to it. This is a vital task and one that has been crucial to the success of the programme.

It is interesting to note in the initial pilot evaluations that, despite some criticisms, 'employers remained unanimous supporters of the programme and described the newly-qualified workers as more confident, mature, innovative and knowledgeable' (Elliot-Cannon and Harbinson, 1995: 16). This description seems to suggest that the challenge of completing a programme which merges two trainings can itself have a developmental impact on those who undertake it. It can be argued that a degree of resourcefulness is needed to manage the dilemmas and change which a joint programme presents to the student. Developing this resourcefulness arguably makes for practitioners who are able to work autonomously and independently in many situations. Certainly the placements on the programme are designed to foster good self-management skills in practice.

Evaluation of the South Bank programme

Evaluation carried out with students has tended to reveal a consensus that the programme is very demanding, and some students have suggested it should be longer in duration. Generally feedback has been positive about the breadth of knowledge covered and about the diversity of practice experience, although some students have wanted more 'statutory'(fieldwork) experience in the branch, either in social work or nursing. Students have expressed the view that learning disabilities was not always given enough attention in the CFP, which was perceived by some to have a more adult nursing focus. They have, however, generally commented favourably on the value of sharing learning with their peers from the other branches of nursing. With regard to support in establishing an 'identity', it has been commented that having a jointly trained member of staff in the team would have been helpful.

The course team undertook a small-scale follow-up research project in 1997 which provided information to the regional health authority on progress with the programme thus far. At that stage only two groups of students had completed the programme, a total of 15 people. In terms of career progression, it was ascertained that of 14 former students the first destinations were as follows: seven had gone to/gone back to work in nursing/health organisations, six of these specialising in learning disabilities; five students had gone into social work posts, one into a disability team, two to children and families teams, one to a hospital discharge team and one to an emergency duty team; and one person had gone into a care management organisation specialising in learning disabilities.

Questionnaires were sent to the former students and their employers regarding the perceived impact of their training on their practice. Students were asked about the value of joint training to their practice and how they had used it. Managers were asked what their organisation had gained from having employed a joint practitioner. There was clear convergence of views in respect of the outcomes of joint training.

A key theme that emerged from the responses was the ability to take a holistic approach. One former student talked about the ability to bridge some of the gaps between services and to co-ordinate service provision from different sources. Another student, who had returned to residential work on completion of the programme, said that 'it was evident to me that the social needs (of residents) were fairly well addressed but the health needs were poorly addressed. I was able to use my experience to bring these to the attention of the relevant individuals and other professionals'. A third student employed as community nurse had been very active in establishing jointly run groups with the local social services department in topics such as health promotion and relationships.

A social services manager observed that 'community care requires agencies to look at the whole person and a joint practitioner may be able to identify needs that a singly trained social worker wouldn't'. Another manager from a nursing team acknowledged that 'although nurses should be able to develop a holistic approach, this can "get lost" in teams where practitioners are all singly trained'. These and other comments appeared to indicate that there was a consensus among respondents that joint training gives a wider range of perspectives on best practice.

Another theme that emerged was that former students appeared to have an understanding of different cultures and language, and that this made multi-disciplinary working easier. One student commented that she had 'found it easy to work with other professionals, having an appreciation of their perspective in assessment'. Another perceived 'an ability to balance and compromise with different professionals' given an understanding of different roles, and a further student spoke of the value of 'understanding the culture differences between health and social care models'. A nurse manager commented that 'singly trained nurses can often see the negative side of social services, but someone also trained is social work will see the positive side before the negative'. Overall, there seemed to be a consensus that increased awareness of other professional contexts, roles and perspectives was a benefit to relationships, and by implication, to working practice.

The third theme that responses revealed concerned a perceived ability to bring additional, complementary skills or perspectives to the context in which the student was working. One former student observed this as an 'ability to offer a perspective that reflects the variety of service provision clients experience'. Another stated that 'working in an almost exclusively nursing environment... joint training has enabled me to consider alternatives which may not have been considered from a strictly nursing perspective'. Correspondingly, the manager of a social services disability team valued employing a social worker who was also a nurse because many of the clients were physically and mentally frail. It was an additional advantage to be able to access the practitioner's nursing skills and knowledge. Equally, the manager of a social services respite care service recognised the benefit of employing a nurse with a strong social perspective. Furthermore, two former students said they had found themselves working in social work settings where there was a need to act on healthcare needs that had previously gone undetected.

Another factor that was mentioned by respondents was the notion of having a 'wider' knowledge base from which to work. One manager commented that the training had given the joint practitioner a 'varied experience, widening concepts in clinical and theoretical knowledge'. In a nursing team, a manager said that the 'inside knowledge' about social services could be passed on to other nursing colleagues. Equally, in a social work environment, the joint practitioner had enabled other staff to 'access information around medical issues, rather than just reading it in a book'.

Conclusion

This chapter has aimed to describe and reflect upon a development in education and training which has the potential to support change in service delivery towards a more integrated approach, in line with expressed public policy. The concept of the joint practitioner is now a familiar one in the field of learning disabilities, and it is to be hoped that this may be one means of ensuring a more holistic approach will be adopted within services, both by individual practitioners and by the teams within which they work. This is not to suggest that these practitioners are better than those who are singly trained, but that they are likely to be *different* in their approach, and this difference may help to create useful change. Given that health and social care needs can be seen as closely interrelated, common sense appears to support the training of practitioners who are competent in both areas. This is particularly relevant to the field of learning disabilities, where the history of approaches has moved from medical to social to health but where none of these models has really provided the holistic support to individuals that they could most benefit from.

Some lessons can be learned from the emergence of joint training which could potentially be applied to other developments in multi-professional learning. These are as follows.

- A competency-based approach can successfully broaden the ability of practitioners to respond effectively to the overlapping health and social dimensions of care.
- This ability to respond can be achieved simultaneously with, and not necessarily at the expense of, the development of specialist practice.
- Education and training grounded in practice partnerships maintains currency and relevance and ensures fitness for purpose and practice.
- Multi-professional learning can help to develop the competencies required for stronger partnership working across traditional professional boundaries.
- In some cases, multi-professional learning may offer the potential for one specialist practitioner to undertake different roles in respect of the same client, thus reducing 'over exposure' to more professionals than is necessary.

References

Barr, H (1998) Competent to Collaborate: Towards a Competency-Based Model for Interprofessional Education, London, *Journal of Interprofessional Care*, **12**(2).

Bartholomew, A, Davis, J and Weinstein, J (1996) *Interprofessional Education and Training. Developing New Models*. London: CCETSW.

Department of Health and Social Security (1971) *Better Services for the Mentally Handicapped*. Command 4683. London: HMSO.

DoH (1998) *Modernising Social Services. Promoting Independence Improving Protection, Raising Standards*. London: Department of Health.

DHSS (1972) *Report of the Committee of Nursing* (Briggs Report), Command 5115. London: HMSO.

Elliot-Cannon, C and Harbinson, S (1995) *Building a Partnership. Cooperation to Promote Shared Learning in the field of Learning Disability*. London: ENB/CCETSW.

ENB (1994) *Creating Lifelong Learners. Partnerships for Care. Guidelines for Pre-registration Nursing Programmes of Education*. London: ENB.

ENB/CCETSW (1995) *Shared Learning. A Good Practice Guide*. London: CCETSW.

Jay Committee (1979) *Report of the Committee of Enquiry into Mental Handicap Nursing and Care*. Command 7468. London: HMSO.

Malin, N (ed.) (1995) *Services for People with Learning Disabilities*. London: Routledge.

Means, R and Smith, R (1994) *Community Care Policy and Practice.* London: Macmillan – now Palgrave.

Mencap (1997) *Prescription for Change.* London: Mencap.

NHSE (1997) *The New NHS Modern Dependable.* London: Department of Health.

NHSE (1998) *Signposts for Success in Commissioning and Providing Health Services for People with Learning Disabilities.* London: Department of Health.

4

Inter-professional Teaching Programme on Normal Labour for Midwifery and Medical Students

Margaret McCarey and Gary Mires

Introduction

Multi-professional education has been widely advocated as an educational strategy. The perceived potential benefits of this approach include the development of the student's ability to share knowledge and skills, enhanced personal and professional confidence, the development of respect between professionals and the encouragement of reflective practice (Areskog, 1994; Goble, 1994; Carpenter, 1995; Pirrie *et al.*, 1998).

Multi-professional teaching is advocated with pre- as well as post-registration students but there is a lack of evaluated research evidence to support this practice (Pirrie *et al.*, 1998, Carpenter, 1995). However, the importance of introducing multi-professional education at an early stage in training has been argued (Horder, 1996).

Multi-professional teaching about the care of women in labour was introduced into the curriculum of the Faculty of Medicine, Dentistry and Nursing, University of Dundee, in January 1998. Prior to this medical and midwifery students were taught the practice and principles of their subject solely by members of their own profession and solely within their professional designation.

This chapter will describe the planning, implementation and evaluation of a programme of teaching on the topic of normal labour to a group of first-year student midwives and third-year medical students within the faculty. Such a teaching programme involving midwifery and medical students learning together had not been attempted within the faculty before this initiative was developed.

The chapter will begin by viewing the initiative in the wider context, namely the transfer of midwifery education into higher education. A detailed description of the inception of the idea will follow together with an explanation of the way the programme was organised and delivered. The methods adopted to evaluate the programme will be included along with a summary of results of the evaluation exercise from a student and staff perspective. The chapter will also address the limitations of the initiative as well as the factors that are considered to have been influential to the success of the programme.

The aim of the programme was to provide a multi-professional learning environment aimed at not only improving knowledge on the topic of normal labour, but also to increase awareness of professional roles. The initiative took place within a faculty with an ongoing commitment to the promotion of multi-professional education as a strategic goal. The stated reasons for this strategy (Faculty of Medicine, Dentistry and Nursing, University of Dundee, internal document 1998) are to:

- provide a richer education for both students and teachers
- develop mutual respect for, and understanding of, other professional groups
- promote greater understanding among students of their own professional roles
- develop the efficient use of shared resources
- promote better preparedness for post-registration work in multi-professional teams
- promote multi-professional research.

Context

The move to higher education by the Fife College of Health Studies and Tayside College of Nursing and Midwifery into the

University of Dundee led to the creation of the School of Nursing and Midwifery within the Faculty of Medicine, Dentistry and Nursing formerly the Faculty of Medicine and Dentistry. The school provides a pre-registration higher education diploma in midwifery programme and has a committed team of midwife lecturers. The established medical curriculum in phase 2 (year 3) on normal labour lasted only three days and comprised clinical skills, integrated teaching boards and a series of lectures, and was about to be supplemented by the newly developed computer assisted learning (CAL) programme. The midwifery curriculum addressed the topic over a period of weeks and activities included lectures, clinical skills, group work and tutorials.

Prior to the merger with higher education there existed a long-standing working relationship between the midwifery lecturers in the school and the obstetricians within the Department of Obstetrics and Gynaecology of the Faculty of Medicine and Dentistry. This relationship and mutual respect contributed greatly to the smooth conduct of the negotiations which preceded the running and facilitation of the programme. On the basis of this aforementioned existing working relationship, an invitation was issued to the midwife lecturers by the obstetricians responsible for the obstetric component of the medical curriculum, to contribute to the creation of a CAL package for medical students on the subject of normal labour.

Whilst initial discussions focused entirely on the development of the CAL programme it soon became apparent that the same programme could be accessed and utilised purposefully by the students of midwifery as both types of students require knowledge of the physiology and management of normal labour. From these discussions the feasibility of developing a wider package of learning centred on normal labour was explored and consequently the possibility of creating a common curriculum to suit midwifery and medical students became the focus of the deliberations.

One of the major obstacles to multi-professional learning is the difficulty in timetabling (Parsell and Bligh, 1998) (see Chapters 1 and 5). However, the window of opportunity presented when it was recognised that the topic of normal labour was scheduled for the same time in both the midwifery and medical curricula. This coinciding of the timetables then provided a real impetus for the development of a programme of multi-professional learning between midwifery and medical students which would incorporate a range of teaching and learning strategies.

The Initiative

The programme hinged on the development of agreed common learning outcomes which were derived from the two curricula and which could be met within the allocated teaching period of two weeks. These outcomes recognised that the requirements of the two groups in terms of knowledge and skills were different and that the midwifery students would go on to address issued in more depth.

The organisers of the programme met regularly to establish mutually acceptable outcomes derived from existing outcomes used by the two schools. Concessions were made on both sides to achieve this goal and this was central to the running of the initiative. These common objectives therefore provided focus and direction to the programme. Areskog (1995) identifies one of the difficulties and constraints of multi-professional education as 'Difficulty in preparing a common core curriculum' (p. 129). In this case the topic was concise and difficulties were not encountered for reasons already alluded to. The common curriculum was arrived at through negotiation, co-operation and a desire to make the programme succeed.

The common objectives incorporated the physiological, psychological and management issues surrounding normal labour and delivery. Also contained within the outcomes were the aspects of role appreciation and relationships between health care professionals involved in the provision of care to the labouring woman.

The common objectives were that at the end of the programme of teaching on labour and delivery the student would be able to:

- demonstrate an understanding of the biochemistry of the onset of labour and the physiology of the stages of labour
- define the stages of labour
- demonstrate a knowledge of the methods of maternal and foetal monitoring in labour

- demonstrate a knowledge of the types of analgesia used in labour
- assess the progress of labour using a partogram and other methods
- understand the mechanisms of normal labour and delivery
- be aware of the psychological aspects of the management of labour
- appreciate the roles and relationship of the health care professionals involved in the provision of care to the labouring woman.

The programme required several shifts of curricular content and reconfiguration of past established timetables. The time allocated to the existing medical curriculum for normal labour could not be extended but it was reconfigured in terms of the established teaching methods used. The midwifery timetable was altered to facilitate this multi-professional learning opportunity by moving subjects traditionally taught before the management of labour, that is, anatomy and physiology. These alterations were made following much debate but in the spirit of co-operation with the will and determination to see the programme succeed. Decisions were also made to use the exercise as a means of exploring the whole notion of multi-professional learning and to evaluate the programme for this purpose using questionnaires. The next phase of the planning involved making decisions about the ways in which the curriculum would be delivered. In order to achieve the learning outcomes it was decided to use a variety of teaching methods to maximise students' learning and understanding.

Teaching/Learning methods

A variety of learning methods were incorporated into the programme as it is recognised that learning is more effective 'when a range of learning methods are offered' (Funnell, 1995: 167). Problem-based Learning (PBL) was adopted as one such learning method. PBL is recognised as being of particular benefit within a multi-professional education context as it fosters a climate of co-operation within a small group of learners (Harden, 1998; Brandon and Majumdar, 1997). PBL replaced all but one of the lectures previously included in the medical curriculum on normal labour. PBL had recently been introduced into the School of Nursing and Midwifery and therefore the midwife lecturers were cognisant of this method of learning having had a series of instruction sessions on this learning strategy.

The other facilitators received staff development on PBL from a member of the medical education department within the University.

Another learning method to be incorporated into the programme was the newly designed interactive CAL programme on the subject of normal labour. The programme took the students about two hours to complete. The obstetricians and midwife lecturers were involved in the review of the CAL programme before the final version was produced.

A two-hour session was designed using integrated teaching boards. (See examples in Appendix 4.1). These boards were designed to present students with clinical and professional issues to consider interactively. Each board required the students to discuss the study material presented, interpret the meaning and reach a consensus on the task set.

This learning method had been used for some years within medical curriculum and was accepted by the midwife lecturers as relevant for midwifery students. Two new boards were designed to take account of the reconfigured learning outcomes, one of which related to professional roles and the other addressing foetal position in labour.

Two-hour sessions in the Clinical Skills Centre provided the students with demonstration and participation in skills surrounding the subject of normal labour. Clinical skills sessions were an established part of both curricula before the programme started as they are perceived as a beneficial medium to enhance learning and the application of theory to practice. Again, agreement was reached by the programme planners regarding the range of skills to be included within the programme.

A study guide was installed on the Web to be accessed by students which provided reference material and a self-assessment section. Students had access to the Web site at times to suit their schedule.

Planning of the programme

The two cohorts of students numbered 180 in total; the mid-wifery students 35 and the medical students 145. Due to the incongruent numbers in each group and in order to evaluate the programme fully by making comparisons between types of education, the total group was divided into eight uni-professional groups comprising medical students and eight multi-professional groups of midwifery and medical students. The numbers in the groups were limited to 10–12 students in order to facilitate PBL. The groups were allocated at random by the planners of the programme. There was a 2:1 medical to midwifery student ratio in the multi-professional groups. From feedback this ratio did not appear to hamper the working of the groups.

The timetable was designed to ensure that the all students had exposure to all types of learning methods during the programme. Personnel were identified to facilitate the 16 PBL groups. These facilitators comprised midwifery lecturers, obstetricians, general practitioners and educationalists. Some of the same personnel were also identified to teach the clinical skills, supervise the integrated teaching boards and assist students in the use of the CAL programme in the computer suite. The planning of the programme was crucial. Communication with staff and students was achieved by use of written timetables and information packs. The securing of suitable accommodation and video recorders for the 16 groups for the PBL sessions was in itself no mean feat. Midwifery and medical students were informed briefly about the programme prior to the Christmas vacations and therefore were prepared to a some extent for this venture on their return.

Delivery of the programme

On the first morning the students assembled and, following a brief introduction to the programme, a lecture on physiology of labour was delivered by a midwife lecturer. Thereafter the students divided into their respective PBL groups and had the first session including the trigger – a video in this case – on normal labour. Over the next three days the students were programmed to attend each of the aforementioned activities, clinical skills,

CAL programme and integrated teaching boards, all of which related to the topic of normal labour. Study time was also written into the programme to enable the students to investigate and collate the information required to fulfil the PBL exercise.

Problem-based learning

The problem-based learning exercise was divided into three separate sessions according to the established principles described by Barrows (1986). Each group, be it uni-professional or multi-professional, began the exercise with a two-hour session during which they were presented with the trigger, a video of a woman in normal labour, and the following question: 'What information do you require in order to provide optimum physical and emotional care for a woman during the first stage of labour?' The group was invited to discuss the video and reach a consensus regarding the information they required to obtain in order to provide optimum care to a woman during the intrapartum period. Having agreed on the distribution of work among the group they had two days before meeting for a review session – again with the facilitator. This session lasted about an hour and reviewed the progress the group had made. The facilitator was present to answer any queries and to guide the group if necessary. The final session was scheduled to last two to three hours and comprised the feedback of information to the whole group by the group in the presence of the facilitator. This session took place during the afternoons of the second week of the programme. This arrangement resulted in each group having a varying length of time to prepare their feedback material. Two facilitators (educationalists) requested the assistance of a 'content expert' at the feedback session to ensure accuracy of information being presented by the students.

Clinical skills

Four clinical skills stations were organised. The skills related to:

- demonstration of a delivery using a delivery pack and a model

- digital vaginal examination in labour – students had the opportunity to practise this skill using anatomical models
- mechanism of labour – students practised this using models following a demonstration and with the use of a handout
- the techniques of donning a sterile gown and surgical gloves – all students practised these techniques following a demonstration.

Students had 30 minutes at each station and rotated around all four. Each station was conducted by a mixture of midwife lecturers and medical colleagues. All sessions were participatory and inter-active allowing for students to practice the skills within their groups.

Integrated boards

Integrated teaching boards comprised of four study boards concerned with clinical problems and professional issues (see Appendix 4.1).

The first board related to the professional roles of midwives and doctors concerning the admission of a woman in labour. Students were set the task of deciding the most appropriate professional to be involved in two separate scenarios. The second board presented the students with information about cardiotoco-graphy and foetal blood sampling. The task of interpreting three examples of each was the focus of this board. The third board gave information relating to the assessment of progress in labour. The task set for students was to comment upon three examples of partograms. The final board involved a knowledge of anatomy and its application to determining foetal position in labour. The groups of students, both multi-professional and uni-professional, worked through all the boards and together discussed the study material presented. A facilitator was present to assist students by clarifying any issues and promoting learning. Following the students' deliberations, feedback was shared with the total group and again this was facilitated by a mixture of midwifery and medical lecturers.

The range of teaching and learning methods utilised proved popular and beneficial with students and lecturers. The variety of methods allowing for dialogue and participation between all concerned.

Evaluation process

Evaluation of the programme was essential. Much discussion surrounded the subject of evaluation and ultimately a decision was made to evaluate the programme in three ways. The planning group was keen to assess the extent to which the students' knowledge changed as a result of the programme. As one of the benefits of multi-professional education is seen to be improved working relationships, it was decided to evaluate the students existing perceptions of the role of the midwife and doctor and assess if those perceptions were altered after the programme. An overall evaluation of the programme was also included in the process.

A knowledge questionnaire was completed at the beginning and the end of the programme. A pre- and post-test was distributed to all 180 students to assess existing and acquired knowledge of labour. The knowledge questionnaire addressed 20 questions which covered questions about basic science, mechanisms of labour and clinical practice. The students were invited to answer the questions 'true/false' or 'don't know'.

An attitude questionnaire which had been developed and piloted by the Centre of Medical Education, University of Dundee, was completed at the beginning and again at the end of the programme. The questionnaire comprised three sections (see Appendix 4.2).

The first section, section A, asked students to rate the responsibility for 21 different clinical tasks. In section B students were asked to rate seven aspects of the provision of information in labour. In sections A and B students were asked which professional was responsible for various activities. These activities related to clinical aspects of care in labour and information giving to women in labour. Students were asked to indicate which activities were 'the midwife's sole responsibility', 'the midwife's the main responsibility', 'the responsibility was shared by doctors and midwives', 'the doctor's main responsibility' and 'the doctor's sole responsibility'. Section C addressed five non labour-related issues covering administrative and managerial duties, for example budgeting, which were not covered in the programme and which acted as control questions. Students were asked to rate these activities by using a five-point scale from 'definitely yes' to 'definitely no' according to whether or not the descriptor best described the role of the midwife or the doctor. Students were also requested to complete an evaluation form relating to the whole programme of education and the learning experience. This questionnaire addressed the issues of multi-professional education, teaching and learning methods, organisation and students' enjoyment of the programme. In addition, the lecturers involved in the programme were also asked to complete a questionnaire to evaluate the total programme.

Evaluation results

Ninety per cent (159/176) of the class completed the pre-course questionnaires and 89 per cent (157/176) completed the post-course questionnaires and student evaluations.

Knowledge questionnaire

The mean number of correct responses on the pre-test for all students was 8.9/20 (95 per cent CI 8.5 to 9.4) compared to 16.0/20 (95 per cent CI 15.7 to 16.4) for the post-course test. On the pre-test, midwifery students scored more highly than the medical students. This finding might be explained by the fact that medical students had had no prior practical experience within the maternity unit whereas the midwifery students had had seven weeks exposure. Both the midwifery and medical students showed a significant increase in the number of correct responses in the post-course test (midwifery students T test 7.1 $p < 0.001$; medical students T test 26.3 $p < 0.001$). The mean number of correct responses on the post-course test was similar for both groups of students.

Attitude questionnaire

Prior to the programme there was significant difference between the midwifery and medical students' perceptions of roles and responsibilities relating to the management of normal labour.

The differences were evident in 14/21 questions asked in section A which focused on clinical activities within a labour ward setting and 6/7 questions asked about the provision of information in section B. Differences in attitudes between students towards their roles were less marked following the programme. Significant differences were found in only 3/21 clinical task questions and in 2/7 of the information provision questions.

Overall, attitudes towards professional roles changes significantly following the programme.

There was an appreciable overall shift in attitude towards a greater midwifery role in care delivery and information giving (Figures 4.1 and 4.2). The shift was more noticeable with the medical students who in general prior to the programme held opinions centred around a shared role between doctors and midwives. There was a significant change in 27/28 questions for the medical students taught in uni-professional groups and in 22/28 questions for medical students taught in multi-professional

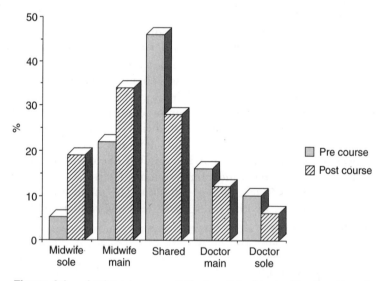

Figure 4.1   Assigned responsibility for clinical tasks (Section A) – all students (*p* < 0.001: chi squared 439.5 pre versus post course)
Source: Reproduced with kind permission from *Medical Teacher*, 1999, **21**(3), 281–85

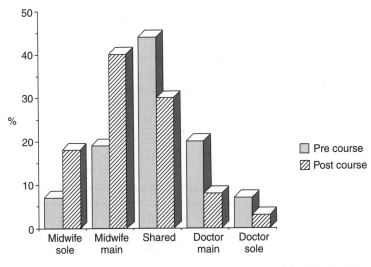

Figure 4.2 Assigned responsibility for information provision (Section B) –
all students (*p* < 0.001: chi squared 245.74 pre versus post course)
Source: Reproduced with kind permission from *Medical Teacher*,
1999, **21**(3), 281–85

groups. Midwifery students significantly changed their views
towards a greater midwifery responsibility in only 4/28 questions.
There was no change in attitudes about the non labour-related
questions in section C by either midwifery or medical students.

Evaluation of the programme

All students expressed positive attitudes towards the programme.
   All midwifery students and 88 per cent of medical students
rated the programme as the same or more useful a learning
activity than other programmes in their curricula. The whole
programme was very much appreciated by the students and the
two cohorts complemented each other in relation to the knowledge they brought to the discussions. Ninety-one per cent of
midwifery students and 83 per cent of medical students felt that
multi-professional teaching programmes should be introduced
into other parts of the curriculum.

The parts of the programme the students found most help-ful were the clinical skills sessions and the integrated teaching boards. The medical students rated PBL less well compared to midwifery students and this finding may reflect the medical students unfamiliarity with the method. Conversely the midwives were less enthusiastic regarding the CAL programme but this finding may be due to them being less familiar with the use of computers.

A large proportion of students were in favour of multi-professional teaching being introduced into other parts of the curricula.

The teaching staff involved were enthusiastic about the approach and are keen to extend multi-professional learning to other areas of the midwifery and medical curricula. Some reservation was expressed about the use of PBL although it was agreed to repeat the programme in the coming academic year.

Limitations

The planning of the programme was very time consuming for the small group involved. The programming was complex as each group required access to all learning activities in a very short period of time. Other midwifery classes had to be adjusted to free up the lecturers to participate in the programme. The programme demanded a high level of commitment from those involved and was very heavy on resources.

Each PBL facilitator was required to be available for three sep-arate sessions, the average time for each session being two hours. The clinical skills sessions were equally intensive on resources requiring eight members of lecturing staff to lead eight groups, through four clinical sessions on two mornings, lasting from 09.00 hours to 13.00 hours. This involved all midwifery lecturers and two obstetricians. The integrated boards sessions numbered four and were each facilitated by two staff, one midwife lecturer and one obstetrician while the CAL programme was supervised by computer experts and a content expert to address knowledge-based questions. The evaluation of the programme produced some interesting data by comparing midwifery and medical student responses as well as multi- and uni-professional group responses.

Although the evaluation made comparisons between multi- and uni-professional groups, the small number of midwifery students precluded the formation of a midwife only group, thus preventing further comparisons.

Keys to success

It is reasonable to conclude that the initiative was a success given the positive evaluation from students and staff.

There are other reasons for the success of the programme. The programme was delivered as an established part of the curriculum in both schools. This was possible because of fortuitous timetabling on this topic in both curricula. The topic of normal labour lends itself to multi-professional teaching, with midwives and doctors working very much as a team in terms of the management of labour. Other successful examples of multi-professional initiatives include those which emphasise such teamwork and relate to professional roles (Wahlstrom *et al.*, 1997; Areskog, 1994). The innovative programme had support at senior level in both schools. No obstacles or barriers were put in the way of the programme proceeding; there was only encouragement and assistance. The success is due in the most part to the efforts of those involved as the initiative was carried out in a spirit of mutual respect and with a will for it to succeed. Staff from the School of Nursing and Midwifery and the School of Medicine worked in a co-operative atmosphere and had very positive expectations. All planning meetings were held jointly to facilitate a feeling of ownership.

The programme organisers explicitly recognised the differences as well as the similarities between the requirements of the two groups of students. This resulted in the development of common objectives which would be achieved in a shared programme, accepting that the midwifery students would require to study the topic in greater depth. The content of the programme and the teaching and learning methods were agreed by both schools, and existing resources and expertise were shared without hesitation. Another major reason for the successful programme lies with the midwifery and medical students who took part in a spirit of co-operation despite their initial anxieties.

Implications for the future

Plans are underway to expand the multi-professional education programmes between midwifery and medical students. Since this programme was completed, discussions have taken place as to the feasibility of developing a programme on antenatal care and aspects of gynaecology. It is also the intention to repeat the programme on normal labour next year.

Conclusion

This chapter has outlined the multi-professional education initiative between first-year diploma midwifery and third-year undergraduate medical students in the University of Dundee.

The constraints which present during the planning phase of a multi-professional education programme are identified by Parsell and Bligh (1998). These constraints include problems with timetabling, huge discrepancies in numbers of students and the different learning methods in place in different departments. Despite these difficulties, all of which were faced while planning this initiative, the programme proved successful, judging by the evaluations of students and staff.

Horder (1996) recommends that multi-professional education begins during students' education programme rather than after qualification in order to pre-empt the formation of negative attitudes towards other professionals. This initiative produced a shift in attitudes about professional roles and evidence from free-text responses suggests that both cohorts of students had more knowledge of the other's responsibilities within a labour ward. Although it is not possible to conclude that positive attitudes will prevail in the minds of the students, Horder's (1996) opinion was reinforced at an evening seminar held by the multi-professional steering group. At this seminar a midwifery and a medical student gave verbal and informal feedback on the programme. They both made very positive comments which contained the clear message that it made perfect sense to learn together when, in future, they would work together when qualified.

The total student cohort evaluated the programme positively and responded well to the learning methods adopted. There appeared to be good interaction between students, and hopefully long-term benefits will result in terms of improved working relationships.

References

Areskog, N H (1994) Multiprofessional Education at the Undergraduate level – the Linköping Model, *Journal of Interprofessional Care*, **8**, 279–82.

Areskog, N H (1995) Multiprofessional Education at the Undergraduate Level. In Soothill, K, Mackay, L and Webb, C (eds), *Interprofessional Relations in Health Care*. London: Edward Arnold.

Barrows, H S (1986) A Taxonomy of Problem Based Learning Methods, *Medical Education*, **20**, 481–6.

Brandon, J E and Majumdar, B (1997) An Introduction and Evaluation of Problem-Based Learning in Health Professions Education, *Family Community Health*, **20**(1), 1–15.

Carpenter, J (1995) Interprofessional Education for Medical and Nursing Students: Evaluation of a Programme, *Medical Education*, **29**, 265–72.

Funnell, P (1995) Exploring the Value of Interprofessional Shared Learning. In Soothill, K Mackay, L and Webb, C (eds), *Interprofessional Relations in Health Care*. London: Edward Arnold.

Harden, R M (1998) AMEE Guide No 12: Multiprofessional Education: Part 1 Effective Multiprofessional Education: A Three Dimensional Perspective, *Medical Teacher*, **20**, 401–7.

Horder, J (1996) The Centre for the Advancement of Inter-Professional Education, *Education for Health*, **9**(3), 397–400.

Goble, R (1994) Multiprofessiona education in Europe. In Leathard, A (ed.), *Going Inter-professional. Working Together for Health and Welfare*. London: Routledge.

Parsell, G and Bligh, J (1998) Interprofessional Learning, *Postgraduate Medical Journal*, **74**, 89–95.

Pirrie, A, Wilson, V, Harden, R and Elsegood, J (1998) AMEE Guide No. 12: Multiprofessional Education: Part 2: Promoting Cohesive Pracice in Health Care, *Medical Teacher*, **20**, 408–15.

Wahlstrom, O, Sanden, I and Hammar, M (1997) Multi-Professional education in the Medical Curriculum, *Medical Education*, **31**, 425–9.

78

Appendix 4.1   Sample integrated teaching boards

Failure to progress in labour can occur due to:
- Faults in the **powers** i.e. failure of adequate uterine activity
- Faults in the **passages** i.e. a small or contracted pelvis
- Faults in the **passenger** i.e. malposition of the vertex (e.g. occipito posterior) or malpresentation (e.g. brow presentation)

These are known collectively as the '3 Ps'

Below are three partograms completed from three different labours.

Partogram I is a partogram demonstrating normal progress in terms of cervical dilatation and descent of the head in association with adequate uterine activity.

Task 1

Study the features of this partogram and compare it with **partograms 2 and 3** which both demonstrate failure to progress.

Comment on the features of the partograms 2 and 3.

Task 2

Using the information given above decide what you consider to be the most likely reason for the failure to progress in partograms 2 and 3, giving reasons for your decision.

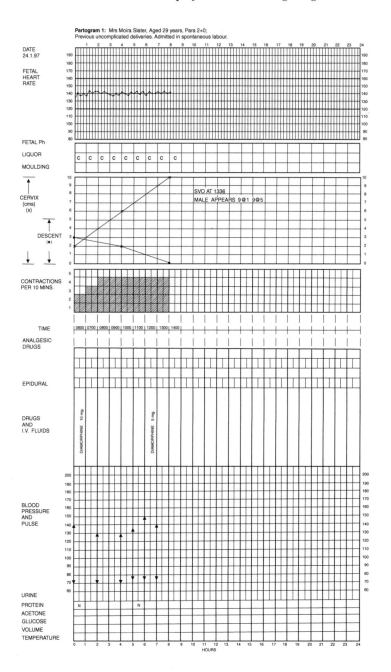

Partogram 1: Mrs Moira Slater, Aged 29 years, Para 2+0;
Previous uncomplicated deliveries. Admitted in spontaneous labour.

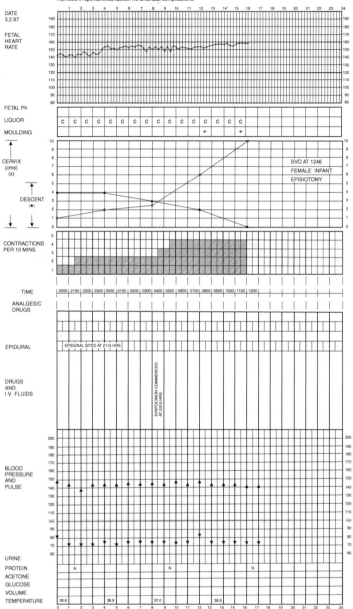

Partogram 2: Mrs Teresa Archer, Aged 22 years, Height 168 cms, Para 0+0;
Admitted in spontaneous labour. No antenatal complications.

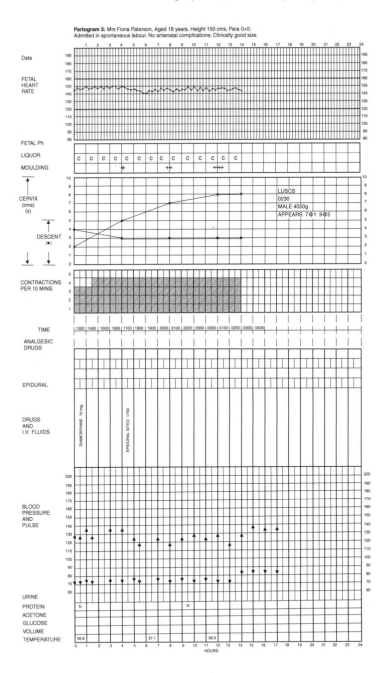

Partogram 3: Mrs Fiona Paterson, Aged 18 years, Height 150 cms, Para 0+0; Admitted in spontaneous labour. No antenatal complications. Clinically good size.

Appendix 4.2   Tasks which students were asked to assign responsibility to in the attitude questionnaire

Section A: Clinical tasks

1. Attending to emotional needs of the woman (fears, worries, anxieties).
2. Attending to the basic physical needs of the mother (hygiene, elimination).
3. Helping women cope their problems (physical, emotional, social).
4. Building up a rapport with the mother.
5. Gaining the trust and confidence of the mother.
6. Liaising with the partners and relatives.
7. Monitoring the woman's condition and progress in labour.
8. Using technical equipment such as foetal heart rate monitors.
9. Prescribing medication e.g. for pain relief.
10. Administering medication.
11. Carrying out minor invasive procedures, e.g. urethral catheterisation, stitching.
12. Carrying out non invasive procedures, e.g. blood pressure.
13. Intravenous cannulation.
14. Administration of IV drugs.
15. Completing forms for diagnostic tests.
16. Acting as the woman's advocate.
17. Assessing the mother and baby's condition.
18. Planning care for the woman.
19. Evaluating the effect of woman's care.
20. Performing a normal delivery.
21. Performing an operative delivery, e.g. forceps, Caesarean section.

Section B: Information provision

22. Explaining to the woman her progress in labour.
23. Explaining to the woman the routine procedures in the labour ward.

24. Explaining the options for delivery.
25. Explaining the options for pain relief.
26. Explaining technical aspects of treatment, e.g. monitoring.
27. Outline possible complications or difficulties with delivery.
28. Breaking bad news, e.g. stillbirth.

Section C: Non-labour descriptors

29. Advises other professions in the healthcare team on physical aspects of care.
30. Advises other professions in the healthcare team on social aspects of care.
31. Holds a senior clinical manager position within the organisation.
32. Controls a budget for a ward or unit.
33. Leads a clinical audit of patient care services.

5

Learning Clinical Skills: an Inter-professional Approach

Maggie Nicol and Mark Chaput de Saintonge

Introduction

The need for greater co-operation and teamworking between healthcare professionals has long been recognised, and the issues and challenges involved have been fully explored in Chapters 1 and 2. Much of the inter-professional activity between nursing and medicine to date has been post-qualification and based in primary healthcare. This chapter describes a short, inter-professional programme in acute care, involving a small number of final-year medical students and newly qualified nurses, and the way in which this was further modified in an attempt to reach larger numbers of participants.

The programme took place in our Interprofessional Skills Centre, a collaborative venture between the School of Nursing and Midwifery and the School of Medicine and Dentistry (Studdy *et al.* 1994). This provides an ideal environment for inter-professional education because it provides a representation of reality without all the demands and stresses of the real clinical setting. It provides a safe environment in which to learn and practise clinical skills and reflect on and learn from clinical experience. It also provides a neutral environment, which is not regarded as belonging to either nursing or medicine but to both. When the project was initially conceived both schools were much smaller than they are today, and were located close to each other and the skills centre. Since that time, both schools have merged with others to become much larger, and have integrated with different universities. Despite these challenges, the Clinical Skills Initiative has proved successful although it has not been possible to achieve all of the original aims.

One of the original aims of the Clinical Skills Initiative was the introduction of inter-professional clinical and communication skills teaching. However, although the areas of overlap between the skills required by each profession and therefore opportunities for shared learning are well recognised, and despite close collaboration between the two schools, it has proved impossible to achieve this in the undergraduate curriculum. A number of reasons have made it difficult to achieve. The large number of students involved (250 medicine and dentistry and 500 nursing and midwifery per annum) are in different universities on geographically distant campuses. The School of Medicine and Dentistry has one intake per year (September) whereas the School of Nursing and Midwifery has two (September and March) which makes it difficult (if not impossible) to co-ordinate timetables so that such teaching occurs at the correct point in the curriculum. Clinical and communication skills require small-group teaching and so there are no economies of scale to be achieved by grouping the two professions together – it simply means that more small groups need to be accommodated at the same time. The nursing students are divided into groups of approximately 20 to 22 students for clinical skills teaching, which means 12 small-group sessions per week for nursing alone. This requires considerable human resources as well as space, equipment, etc.

Despite our best efforts and many hours spent poring over timetables looking for opportunities, it was reluctantly accepted that it would not be possible to accommodate or provide the resources needed to support inter-professional skills teaching within the current undergraduate/pre-registration curricula. Furthermore, even if these issues were overcome, there was the additional problem that the cohort of nursing students that commence in March each year would have no matching group of medical students. These problems are not unique and similar issues have been reported by others attempting inter-professional initiatives (for example, Carpenter, 1995a; Goble, 1991). Although it is considered desirable to introduce inter-professional learning early, that is before stereotypical attitudes have time to develop

(Areskog, 1988; Carpenter, 1995b), as this was not possible other options were examined. This led us to develop the programme for a small group of newly qualified nurses and final-year medical students.

Inter-professional clinical skills programme

The definition of inter-professional education adopted by the Clinical Skills Initiative is 'interprofessional education involves learning with and from each other'. Thus it was important to ensure that the programme was more than simply students of medicine and nursing in the same room being taught together: it must provide opportunities for 'learning with and from each other'. Seven medical students in their final year on their senior medical attachment and seven staff nurses were recruited. Choosing newly qualified rather than student nurses had one huge advantage: there was only one timetable to contend with. The nurses were able to be flexible and only required the permission of their manager to be able to attend. The manager was approached personally and persuaded of the benefits of allowing them to attend. This was agreed, despite the fact that it meant losing a member of staff, who often had to be replaced by bank or agency staff. The nominated staff nurses were then contacted by letter, giving brief details of the programme and details of timing, venue, etc. Registry identified and notified the medical students.

The programme originally comprised four half-day sessions, one per week for four weeks. The medical students were on their senior medical attachment and the nurses were all recruited from the medical directorate. The selection of nurses and medical students from the one clinical specialty was deliberate so that the scenario, which provided the main focus of the programme, could be relevant to their clinical experience and likely to result in more effective learning (Knowles, 1990; MacLeod and Farrell, 1994). It was also hoped that the participants would meet each other in the course of their work and develop better working and learning relationships. The programme was led by senior lecturers from each school, both of whom had experience in the relevant area of practice and a particular interest in inter-professional education. For the first programme, a GP, clinical nurse specialist and communication skills teachers were also involved. The original programme was extremely successful and has been reported elsewhere (Freeth and Nicol, 1998). However, it was expensive in terms of teaching, and the design meant that only extremely small numbers of students (seven staff nurses and seven medical students) could attend. This led to changes in an attempt to involve more students.

The programme structure

The original programme was reduced in length from four half-days to one whole day. This had the advantage that we were able to run it more frequently and, by increasing the numbers to 20 per day (ten senior medical students and ten nurses) we were able to offer it to more students. It also overcame problems of attendance experienced by the nurses, who had difficulty avoiding clashes with night duty for the four weeks. The disadvantage was that there was less 'social' time, during which participants talked and shared experiences informally. The day began with brief introductions and the group was then divided into separate professions to discuss the clinical scenario. One of two scenarios is used each day. This is to provide some variety and to prevent boredom on the part of the organisers, but both are designed to cover similar clinical and communication skills. One scenario is a newly admitted patient with an ulcer on his foot and cellulitis, who is found to have insulin-dependent diabetes. The other is a patient admitted following a cerebro-vascular accident resulting in left-sided hemiplegia and hemi-sensory loss, who is unable to swallow and has a chest infection (see Figure 5.1). The scenarios have been chosen because they represent typical cases that students are likely to meet in almost any ward but particularly in an acute medical ward.

The day is facilitated by the senior lecturer for clinical skills in nursing, and the director of clinical skills in medicine, who is a physician. They facilitate the whole day together to promote the concept of inter-professional teamworking. To start the day the students are divided into two separate professional groups and each group is facilitated by the appropriate senior lecturer. They are then given the scenario and asked to identify (on a flip

---

Patient scenario 1

Your patient is a 67-year-old man who has been admitted at the request of his GP. For seven days he has been troubled by an ulcer on his right first toe which has gradually been increasing in size. The ulcer developed after he dropped a saucepan on his foot and there is now swelling around the ulcer and redness spreading up the foot and lower leg. His GP has diagnosed ascending cellulitis, noting that he is pyrexial with a temperature of 38.7°C. He has also found that the blood glucose is elevated (23 mmol/L). The patient confirms that he has been excessively thirsty for several months and that this has been accompanied by polyuria, nocturia and weight loss of about 1 stone. He currently weighs 63 kg.

There is no relevant past medical history and no family history of diabetes. He is a widower who lives alone in a one-bedroom flat; he has three children, two of whom live close by. He smokes 10–15 cigarettes a day and drinks the occasional sherry. His GP commenced oral antibiotics 24 hours previously; he is taking no other medication.

On arrival in the ward he is pyrexial, drowsy but very co-operative, and has a blood glucose of 17–28 mmol/L.

Patient scenario 2

Your patient is a 65-year-old married woman who collapses suddenly at home. When her husband finds her she is semi-conscious, aphasic and unable to use her right side. An examination by her GP confirms that she has sustained a left cerebral hemisphere CVA with a right hemiparesis and hemi-sensory loss. In addition, the GP notices that she has injured her shin and a deep ulcerated laceration is present.

The patient is referred for hospital admission. Her husband, daughter and son accompany her to hospital.

Figure 5.1   Clinical scenarios used in the inter-professional study

chart) the care the 'patient' requires and which profession(s) should be responsible for each aspect. This activity is designed to formulate a plan of care for the patient (which provides the framework for the rest of the day) and identify the degree of overlap or shared responsibility between the two professions. It also serves to enable the groups to get to know each other because, although the medical students are likely to know each other relatively well, the nurses may not know each other at all. During this activity the groups begin to relax and share knowledge and experience. The two groups then come together to consider the two action plans. This serves to highlight the similarity and level of agreement between the two groups, but differences, although small, are also important in that they also illustrate the different focus of the two professions and the importance of working together for the benefit of the patient. The different approaches of the two groups were summed up by one medical student who commented 'the nurses have admitted a person, we have admitted a foot!'.

The rest of the day is devoted to discussion, demonstration and practise of the skills required to implement the action plan, setting the various skills in the context of inter-professional patient care and teamwork. This begins with physical assessment of the patient and then intravenous cannulation using model arms. The cannulation technique is demonstrated using a video programme and the medical students, who already have this skill, then teach and supervise the nurses, providing suggestions and tips for successful cannulation from their own experience. Coffee is then provided before the group is divided into four inter-professional groups with two or three nurses and two or three medical students in each. These groups remain together for the rest of the day.

The next activity is prescribing antibiotics, analgesics and intravenous fluids. The groups are provided with prescription charts, pencils, erasers and the *British National Formulary*. The medical students have knowledge of the organisms likely to be present in the foot ulcer or causing the chest infection, and the nurses have knowledge of how this should be prescribed and how it should be administered. Some very interesting discussions developed with nurses arguing against the use of intravenous antibiotics when it was not deemed necessary or, where there was a choice, choosing an antibiotic that required administration only twice a day instead of four times, to reduce the demand on nurses time. The medical students were able to share their knowledge of pathology and pharmacology and the nurses their knowledge of prescribing and management of intravenous therapy. There was also a good deal of discussion regarding the use of the 'prn' and 'once only' sections of the prescription chart, with nurses giving practical advice about how to make sure that these are not overlooked by the nurses on the ward. A plenary session allowed the groups to share their ideas and discuss the merits or disadvantages of the various drugs suggested, and the facilitators were able to ensure that they had arrived at the 'correct' answers.

For the next activity the 'patient' suffers a cardiac arrest. This leads to discussion about the likely causes and interpretation of cardiac rhythms and then, working in interprofessional pairs, the group practise ward-based resuscitation skills. Their efforts are successful and the 'patient' is transferred to the intensive care unit. This is followed by discussion in inter-professional groups about 'not for resuscitation' orders and how to talk to the patient's family. The groups were asked to consider who should talk to the family, where they should talk to them and what the family is likely to want to know. All groups agreed that it would be better if the nurse and doctor spoke to the family together, so that they can support each other and know what has been said, although they recognised why this was not always possible. The nurses in particular commented that they found it hard when they did not know what patients and their families had been told, especially if the family appeared to have misunderstood what had been said. This led to discussion about how to avoid giving false hope and making sure that the family understood what was being said by the avoidance of euphemisms, etc.

The first session of the afternoon was devoted to clinical skills practice. In the same inter-professional groups the participants rotate around a number of 'stations' designed to address a number of clinical skills relevant to the scenario. Each is designed so that the nurses teach the medical students or vice versa. For example, the nurses were able to teach the medical students skills such as blood glucose monitoring and how to prepare an intravenous infusion, and medical students were able to teach the nurses how to perform venepuncture and ophthalmoscopy. The facilitators remain accessible but do not intervene unless asked to do so by the group or if inaccurate information is being given. The scenarios are designed to ensure that a range of the clinical skills performed by both nurses and doctors will be required to manage the 'patient'. This has the advantage that the skills are seen in the context of inter-professional patient care rather than simply a list of skills. It also leads to discussion about who should perform these skills. Lack of clarity can lead to conflict and/or confusion, and patient care suffers if everyone assumes that it is part of someone else's role. It is hoped that discussion of the issues involved will lead to a better understanding of each other's perspective. The following skills are addressed during this session:

- intravenous cannulation and application of the dressing
- venepuncture
- CVP measurement
- preparation of an intravenous infusion
- use of an intravenous infusion pump
- ophthalmoscopy
- blood glucose monitoring (finger prick)
- arterial blood gases
- ECG recording.

The day ends with discussion about discharge planning. In the same inter-professional groups the students discuss issues such as what GPs, district nurses, etc. need to know; how this should be communicated, what other agencies might be involved and how these services are organised.

Discussion

The evaluations were very positive, with all participants saying that they had enjoyed the day and felt that they had benefited by attending. However, it soon became clear that the aims of the programme were different for the organisers and the participants. As far as the participants were concerned, they had been invited to attend to develop their clinical skills. Indeed, this was used to attract them in the first place. However, the aim of the programme as far as the organisers/authors were concerned, was to improve working relationships through better communication and a better understanding of each other's role. The two are not incompatible but it would be quite easy to achieve one at the expense of the other or fail to achieve either. For example, learning intravenous cannulation is probably most efficiently achieved in un-professional groups where the instructor is familiar with the students, their previous knowledge and their learning needs. If the group is inter-professional some learning about each other's profession may occur, but there is a danger that students may leave having gained a better understanding of each other's role but unable to cannulate, or vice versa. Where one group has the skill and the other does not, successful inter-professional teaching and learning can occur, but this inevitably requires additional curriculum time.

The clinical skills component of the course provided a vehicle to attract participants and an opportunity to gain a better understanding of each other's role. In the first course we were successful and evaluations contained comments such as 'it makes you appreciate what nurses do' and 'I have gained a better understanding of the role of house officers and the importance of working together'. However, although both groups felt that they had gained a lot, neither actually went away equipped with new skills. Although the nurses gained insight and some practical experience during the course, they did not have sufficient time to become proficient in skills such as venepuncture and IV cannulation that were new to them. They still needed to attend additional training before expanding their role to include these skills. Despite this, all the nurses who attended felt that the increased knowledge and understanding of the skills covered meant that they were better able to care for patients. Most of the medical students had previously learnt most of the skills covered but did comment that the programme helped them to see the skills within the context of patient care and also to clarify uncertainties.

Thus, as a means of teaching a range of new clinical skills to newly qualified staff nurses and senior medical students, such a course is probably not effective. However, as a means of helping the participants refine and develop existing skills and increase their understanding of the role of another healthcare professional, such a programme appears to have potential. The problem remains, however, that although successful, such programmes can only ever accommodate small numbers of students. It was recognised that if the positive outcomes were ever to be achieved on a large scale, programmes need to be developed that can be delivered outside of the skills centre by many different facilitators.

Clinical governance

'A First Class Service' outlines the Government's quality agenda for the NHS (Department of Health, 1998) at the centre of which is clinical governance. Key elements of this approach include: the adoption of an evidence-based approach, implementation of systems for increased accountability, and increased clinical performance. Underpinning this new quality agenda is the need for clinicians to work closer together in a more co-ordinated fashion. In particular, information sharing, networking and teamwork are all required to forge and then maintain effective inter-professional relationships. A recent survey found that practitioners leading the implementation of clinical governance in their clinical areas considered collaboration and teamwork as key elements (Hayward *et al.* 1999).

Clinical governance provided the vehicle for our next enterprise, a series of three inter-professional sessions for 25 staff nurses and 25 pre registration house officers (PRHOs) in a large London teaching hospital. The sessions took place in the autumn by which time the house officers had had two to three months to settle into their role. The sessions each lasted 90 minutes and took place at lunchtime once a week for three consecutive weeks (lunch is provided to encourage attendance!). Nurse managers were invited to nominate staff nurses to attend. The lunchtime slot was chosen partly because the PRHOs already have sessions at this time each week, and also because it meant that the nurses could be spared from the ward during the afternoon overlap of shifts and would not need to be replaced by agency nurses. This is an important consideration in NHS trusts that are subject to severe financial constraints and the need to make savings.

The focus of each session was a clinical issue that hospital data and anecdotal evidence suggested might be improved through interprofessional collaboration:

1. pain management and prescribing
2. IV therapy and drug administration including the use of IV pumps and syringe drivers
3. Discharge planning.

The sessions took place in a seminar room on the main hospital site with sufficient space to allow participants to work in interprofessional groups. It is important that the venue is close to the wards to enable easy access by those carrying bleeps. Trigger questions are used promote discussion and encourage the participants to work together using each other's knowledge to address the problem. Clinical experts from both professions were present to facilitate the feedback from the groups, add specialist information and correct any misconceptions.

Evaluation of the first series of sessions was through questionnaires and telephone interviews six weeks later. The questionnaire evaluations were extremely positive. All involved (including facilitators and clinical experts) found it enjoyable and felt that addressing these issues in an inter-professional forum added to the experience. The follow-up interviews were equally encouraging. Participants felt they were working together in a more co-ordinated and collaborative fashion. For example, one house officer noted that he now liaised more frequently with nursing staff over discharge planning. Similarly, one of the staff nurses pointed out that she now offered help to doctors when they were setting up IV pumps because discussion in the sessions had highlighted that they had little opportunity to learn how to use them.

The series of three sessions is being repeated, this time with the inclusion of ward pharmacists. Their close involvement in all of the topics discussed was highlighted by the participants who felt that their participation in future sessions would be helpful. The enthusiastic response from all involved has helped convince nurse managers to allow more nurses to attend and discussion with senior pharmacists has been equally positive.

Such an approach seems to have the potential to improve teamwork, and ultimately patient care, by promoting a better understanding of each other's role and contribution to the multidisciplinary team. This initiative was possible because the facilitators meet regularly in order to manage the interprofessional skills centre. Inter-professional initiatives are often frustratingly slow and many ideas wither and die through lack of progress. Having an inter-professional venture such as the Skills Centre Initiative means that there is regular dialogue between the two schools and a real commitment to inter-professional learning. Additional topics for discussion will be piloted next year and, if found to be equally successful, course materials (such as co-ordinator and facilitators packs) will be developed to enable this programme to be 'rolled out' and delivered to much larger numbers of clinical staff working in the NHS.

The programme described above has overcome some of the constraints and problems encountered when attempting to initiate inter-professional activities. The emphasis on clinical governance means that all involved can see the relevance to their everyday practice and managers are more likely to be supportive. The costs are low, requiring only the provision of a light lunch for the participants and a few written scenarios/triggers. Teaching aids and clinical equipment such as IV pumps are usually readily available and most hospitals have a suitable room somewhere. By targeting newly qualified nurses and doctors, the programme is addressing the needs of the two groups who work most closely together in hospital wards and the two groups who need most to understand each other's contribution to the multidisciplinary team. By planning a programme that is simple in design and can be rolled out to a number of different hospitals, it should be possible to reach most if not all of the PRHOs and newly qualified staff nurses, and others in the multi-professional team. Inter-professional study days such as that described earlier in this chapter may be very successful and enjoyable for all concerned, but they will have little impact if only tiny numbers of health professionals can participate. It is hoped that the programme planned here will eventually overcome that problem.

References

Areskog, N-H (1988) The need for multiprofessional health education in undergraduate studies, *Medical Education*, **22**, 251–2.

Carpenter, J (1995a) Implementing community care. In: Soothill, K, MacKay, L and Webb, C (eds), *Interprofessional relations in health care*. London: Edward Arnold.

Carpenter, J (1995b) Doctors and nurses: stereotypes and stereotype change in interprofessional education, *Journal of Interprofessional Education*, **9**(2) 151–61.

Department of Health (1998) *A First Class Service: Quality in the NHS*. London: Stationery Office.

Freeth, D and Nicol, M (1998) Learning clinical skills: an interprofessional approach, *Nurse Education Today*, **18**, 455–61.

Goble, R (1991) Keeping alive intellectually, *Nursing*, **4**(33), 19–22.

Hayward, J, Rosen, R, Dewar, S (1999) Thin on the ground, *Health Service Journal*, 26 August.

Knowles, M (1990) *The adult learner: a neglected species*. (4th edn), Houston, Texas: Gulf Publishing.

Macleod, M and Farrell, P (1994) The need for significant reform: a practice-driven approach to curriculum, *Journal of Nursing Education*, **33**(5), 208–14.

Studdy, S Nicol, M and Fox-Hiley, A (1994) Teaching and learning clinical skills, Part 1: Development of a multidisciplinary skills centre, *Nurse Education Today*, **14**, 177–85.

6

A Perspective of Shared Teaching in Ethics

Cecilia Edward, Ann Roberts and June Small

Introduction

At the University of Dundee, the School of Nursing and Midwifery offers a three-year diploma programme, whilst the School of Medicine provides a five-year medical undergraduate programme of study. During their training the students undertaking these programmes have three collaborative meeting points for shared teaching in ethics at junior, intermediate and senior. At present, the School of Nursing and Midwifery has two intakes per year in March and September. The September intake is involved with the ethics sessions at junior and senior levels, and the March intake at the intermediate level.

The rationale for introducing collaboration meeting points within each student programme was directed towards encouraging professional relationships in health care. To this end a global aim was formulated:

- to enable the student, through the process of shared teaching in ethics, to develop personal/professional ethical and moral reasoning to enhance user and patient care.

The key

Rodgers (1994) states that the provision of high standards of care within the health service is achieved when all professionals involved in patient care collaborate towards a shared common goal. However, it is often the norm that healthcare professionals have been socialised into their future perceived roles within a traditional uni-professional educational process Mackay *et al.* (1995). Once qualified, despite working together, these professionals may not be able to identify, or be sensitive to, the rationale behind care strategies suggested by other members of the multi-professional team. In essence, they may not fully appreciate or understand the views of other professionals in the decision-making process.

Inherent within team decisions, which should ideally encompass collective and communitarian views, there co-exists a degree of 'cultural individualism' (Platt, cited in Casto and Julie, 1994). This, it could be argued, has the potential to jeopardise the delivery of high-quality care for which the team are responsible and accountable. Platt (1994: 4) also suggests that in many instances 'we do not know how to work as a team... how to think as a team.' McKeal *et al.* (1998: 65) advances this notion by stating that the inconsistencies which frequently occur between professional carers 'may stem directly from the separate educational streaming that occurs in each of the health care disciplines'.

These findings promote the argument for shared learning, in the form of multi-professional and inter-professional collaboration meeting points during student training (Ytrehus, 1993; Ekeli, 1996). This indeed, may be the key to the way forward for positive relationships and outcomes in patient care situations.

The ideal

In the early 1990s the then College of Nursing and Midwifery and the School of Medicine at the University of Dundee recognised the importance of the concept of inter-professional learning for healthcare students and decided that future patient care and professional relationships could be enhanced by shared teaching between nursing, midwifery and medical students.

It was postulated that, if the students met during their training to discuss a topic relevant to both student programmes, a 'bonding' process would be initiated. By meeting each other during the theoretical part of their course, the students would have the opportunity to identify and appreciate different points of view related to healthcare issues. In addition, it was believed that the students would also have the opportunity to begin to interact as a team and to recognise and respect the importance of individual and collective autonomy. Forbes and Fitzsimons (1993: 2–3) suggest that the recognition of these principles by members of the health team increases the potential for 'consultation, collaboration, holistic team autonomy and harmony in practice'. This justified the proposal of a pilot study to examine the concept of shared teaching, with the anticipated strengths outweighing its weaknesses.

The challenge for the college and the university was to identify an educational approach which would allow the students to flourish in a 'culture of collaboration' (de Tournay, 1994).

The area of ethics was elected as the topic for shared learning and teaching. There were several reasons for choosing this subject. In the first instance, it was common to both curricula. In addition, due to the advances in medical knowledge and technology, healthcare professionals are required to be more receptive and sensitive to ethical issues at both a macro and micro level.

The seminar format was established as the most appropriate learning and teaching strategy for a discussion related to ethics. This method not only generates a rich cross-fertilisation of different personal/professional points of view related to situations in healthcare, it also gives the students the opportunity to identify the importance of communication skills and appreciate the complexities of group dynamics in a multi-professional setting. Therefore, to have the opportunity to meet during their training to examine and analyse the complexities of moral aspects of patient care appeared desirable (Edward and Preece, 1999).

In the 'real' world of healthcare, nurses, midwives and doctors often have to make difficult ethical decisions concerning what is in the patient's best interests. Ideally, this should be achieved through 'teamwork' 'team thinking' 'team respect' and 'team decision making', culminating in a combined positive good for the delivery of patient care. However, Peter and Gallop (1994) suggest that variations in professional value systems may present conflicting opinions when considering what action will have the best consequence for the patient. This argument is reinforced by Holm (1997), who found that in some instances doctors believed that differences in moral beliefs and professional opinions could create barriers to the making of reasoned ethical decisions. Therefore the whole notion of the shared teaching venture was to challenge the traditional uni-professional education of nursing, midwifery and medical students, and to address the problems as stated by Peter and Gallop (1994), and Holm (1997). Nurses, midwives and doctors work with each other and, as WHO (1988) suggests, perhaps they should begin to learn together.

Meeting and collaborating as students could be the first step towards a lifelong process of professional learning and caring: the ideal way forward.

The process towards the Ideal

In the autumn of 1992 senior management within the College of Nursing and Midwifery and the School of Medicine decided that measures should be taken to implement the shared teaching venture. It was agreed that a small-scale study should be carried out.

The first step in the process was to identify two co-ordinators who would initiate the pilot study and explore the possibility of the potential for shared teaching to be incorporated into both student programmes. In the spring of 1993 a nursing lecturer from the College of Nursing and Midwifery and a clinician from the School of Medicine, both experienced in the teaching of ethics within their respective programmes, were requested to take the idea forward.

A small steering group of professionals with academic and clinical credibility comprising two clinicians, two nursing lecturers, a midwifery lecturer and a philosopher was established. The group met on several occasions to determine and agree the aims, expected outcomes and content of the course.

The pilot study focused on a cohort of 68 student volunteers. To prevent role confusion the students selected were not in their first year and therefore had acquired considerable professional identity prior to interacting with other healthcare students. McKiel *et al.* (1988) and Casto and Julie (1994) identify this as an important point for consideration. They suggest that when approaching the topic of ethics, students should have a grasp of their own beliefs, values and professional value systems.

As the pilot study proved popular with both students and facilitators the decision was made that the short course should be identified as the first collaboration meeting point for a junior level of shared teaching in ethics for all nursing, midwifery and medical students.

In 1994 the College of Nursing and Midwifery was awarded a commendation by the King's Fund Partnership Trust for the shared teaching initiative. The award provided both the motivation and stimulus to continue with the development of the venture.

September 1996 saw the merger of the College of Nursing and Midwifery into the Faculty of Medicine and Dentistry. This important development strengthened the idea of shared teaching. Further collaboration meeting points in ethics, at intermediate and senior levels, were identified for 1997.

At present the co-ordinators meet frequently to monitor the quality of these sessions. In addition, the steering group meets approximately once or twice a year to review the three short courses.

In 1997 the steering group invited the facilitators and students who had taken part in the courses to share their opinions and experiences. This meeting now occurs on an annual basis.

The picture

To take the pilot study forward into the three levels of shared teaching the co-ordinators and steering group required vision, creativity, patience and respect for each other (respect in the sense of recognising the contribution of all members and identifying each other as equals).

The following core issues are related to the aims, learning outcomes, educational strategies, and teaching tools (packages and scenarios) of each level.

Aims and learning outcomes

Junior level. Healthcare Ethics

The overall aim of this level is to enable the students to develop an understanding of ethics and its relevance to healthcare within a shared learning environment.

All the students taking part are in their second year with the main focus under discussion being the moral and ethical issues inherent within healthcare settings. A collaboration meeting point at this early stage of their training allows the students to:

- explore, together, the beliefs, attitudes and values of other healthcare professionals
- explore ethical concepts inherent within ethical relationships
- appreciate the need to explore ethical issues in the shared learning environment
- utilise the learning situation to enhance communication in professional relationships
- participate in inter-professional group activities.

Intermediate level. Inter-professional relationships in healthcare

The overall aim of this level is to enable the students to develop skills of decision making in relation to moral and professional issues.

The medical students are in the third year of their course, whilst the nursing and midwifery students are at the end of their second year of training. Therefore, at this stage, both groups of students have had the opportunity to identify their own respective professional boundaries. A collaboration meeting point at this stage of their training allows the students to:

- utilise moral reasoning and ethical sensitivity to analyse ethical issues inherent within healthcare
- recognise individual differences in the ability to appreciate morally sensitive issues

- act with other group members to justify the groups' conclusion to ethical problems using a decision making process.

Senior level. Ethics, professional issues and law

The overall aim of this level is to enable the students, through the process of shared learning, to appreciate the ethical, professional and legal dimensions within the multi-professional team.

The medical students taking part are in their fifth year. The shared teaching course takes place during a three week preparation for their role as junior house officers. The nursing and midwifery students are in their third year. A collaboration meeting point at this stage of their training allows the students to:

- differentiate between the rights of self and others
- appreciate the rights of self and others
- analyse critically the relationships and tensions within the multi-disciplinary team
- appraise the moral dilemmas inherent within healthcare ethics
- analyse critically the role of the autonomous practitioner in choosing the best alternatives in adverse conditions.

Management of student numbers

Three factors influence the number of students taking part in shared teaching, namely admissions to the faculty; attrition rates; and student attendance. Overall the size of the student population ranges from approximately 280 to 350.

As the junior and intermediate levels involve small-group work, this dictated that two cohorts of students were formed for these sessions: sections A and B. Each section was subdivided into eight to ten mixed groups, each of which consisted of 16 to 20 students. Section A have ethics on day X whilst section B are allocated to private study. The situation is then reversed on day Y.

The senior level takes place in a lecture theatre which can accommodate a large student population.

Educational strategy

The seminar format for the junior level involves small groups of students meeting to discuss hypothetical case studies related to issues of truth telling, informed consent and confidentiality. These topics were selected as they would parallel situations students would encounter when working within healthcare settings.

The importance of selecting 'everyday' patient-centred dilemmas to which students are able to relate, and not 'tip-of-the-iceberg' (Seedhouse, 1988) topical moral issues, is an established procedure in ethics instruction (Krawczyk and Kudyma, 1978; Holm, 1997).

Each session lasts for two hours and is facilitated by a nursing/midwifery lecturer from the School of Nursing and Midwifery and a clinician/lecturer from the School of Medicine.

At the intermediate level each group of students is further subdivided into mixed groups of four to five students. They are instructed to analyse a healthcare dilemma and then present their findings to the greater group. This style of learning places the students in a situation which can promote their 'thinking through' a problem in a safe environment. Each session is facilitated by a nursing/midwifery lecturer from the School of Nursing and Midwifery and a clinician/lecturer from the School of Medicine.

The senior level differs from the two previous short courses in that it consists of two separate three-hour sessions. These sessions involve a *mélange* of teaching and learning styles: didactic, buzz groups, debate and a panel discussion. These versatile teaching methods encourage lively and open debate.

The first session encompasses the domain of 'Resuscitation – who decides?' and the second is related to the 'Rights and wrongs of end-of-life issues'. These topics assist the students to identify and analyse critically the moral, professional and legal aspects of resuscitation and end-of-life issues, and the concepts of caring, compassion and humanism within a holistic approach to patent care.

Lecturers and experts from many disciplines participate in this last stage of shared teaching in ethics. It is hoped in future to include students from other faculties to further the concept of multi-professional learning.

Learning and teaching tools

All three levels use some form of case study methodology (Figure 6.1). Many of the case studies utilised were adapted from real-life dilemmas experienced by qualified members of staff, others were taken from texts or created by those lecturers/clinicians involved in the venture. This notion is reinforced by Holm (1997: 143) who suggests that the study of ethics should concentrate on the 'ethical problems of health care professionals'. Indeed, the usefulness of case studies as a teaching tool and learning source is well documented (Self *et al.*, 1989); Vitz, 1990; Mitchell *et al.*, 1992).

Junior level

John is a 24-year-old mechanic who has been involved in an accident at work. On admission to the accident and emergency unit he is unconscious and is in a state of shock. Apparently John has received a blow to the abdomen from a moving crane and the doctor believes that he may have internal bleeding. An intravenous infusion is set up and whole blood is administered. His condition is stabilised. and the peripheral infusion is kept patent with normal saline.

John regains consciousness, and as he looks around him, becomes aware that he is receiving an intravenous infusion. 'What is that you are giving me?' he asks the nurse. She replies that it is some fluid to keep him hydrated and that there is a possibility that he may require an operation to remove his spleen. She informs him that the doctor will be to see him shortly to explain everything to him. 'Its OK about the op., but I can't take a blood transfusion you know, because I am a Jehovah's Witness.' At that moment the doctor enters the room.

Intermediate Level

A patient is examined by a healthcare professional. Later, the patient, who asks to speak to an other healthcare professional, alleges that the examination was more intimate and prolonged than anticipated. Not wishing to be seen as a trouble maker the patent pleads for the matter to be kept confidential. Adapted from Wall; (1993)

Senior Level

Should age determine whether or not to start or continue cardiopulmonary resuscitation?

Figure 6.1   Sample case studies/statements

Prior to the delivery of the junior and intermediate levels information in the form of a package is provided to both facilitators and students. This package, containing aims, learning outcomes and ground rules, is sent out to the facilitators several weeks before the session. The reason for this plan of action is the importance of the facilitators meeting several days or weeks in advance to discuss the content of the package and agree on the process outcomes. This is paramount to the promotion of harmony between the facilitators and the success of the ethics course. The students receive the package immediately prior to the session. This allows for spontaneous individual opinions to be expressed, thus creating a springboard for further, in-depth, diverse ethical discussion.

The learning environment in which the group sessions take place is important. Ideally, it must be sensitive to the personal/ professional feelings and experiences of those present. To create this sense of security ground rules must to be negotiated. These rules include issues such as sensitivity and respect for individual points of view, acknowledgement of the right to self-expression, and confidentiality. It is also advisable that there should only be two facilitators, and consequently observers are not permitted to the session.

Reality challenges

In relation to the progress of the shared teaching venture it cannot be denied that the process has been long and often torturous. However, despite the overall success of the three levels several problems remain, some of which may never be resolved.

Issue 1. Collaboration meeting points

Although the shared teaching takes place in established months of the year, there remains difficulty in matching the sessions to the respective timetables. Both student programmes are dynamic and do not remain static; therefore the time identified as suitable in year X may not be applicable the following year. Over the years this issue has required considerable understanding and tolerance between the co-ordinators and programme leaders from both schools.

Action
Negotiations to accommodate each level take place six months before each course begins.

Issue 2. Classroom availability

The physical environment is an important issue for the junior and intermediate levels as they are required to work in small groups. To find eight to ten suitable rooms for the first two levels is problematic. Many of the rooms in the School of Nursing and Midwifery are too small or are frequently booked for other courses. In the Medical School the classrooms are often unsuitable due to their design, location and size. Student and facilitators evaluations have identified this as an issue, for example, 'room full of equipment'; 'large area had been partitioned'; 'could hear other class going on'.

Action
Identification of suitable rooms has been established. Where possible, rooms are booked ahead of time with each school providing four to five classrooms.

Issue 3. Facilitator availability

In tandem with the issue of classroom accommodation is the problem of facilitator availability for the junior and intermediate levels – these small group sessions require to be facilitated by nursing/midwifery lecturers and clinicians/lecturers.

The initial pilot study identified that student knowledge benefited from the presence of two facilitators who had expertise in nursing/midwifery and medicine. This concept of joint teaching is now an established practice for both, junior and intermediate levels. Ideally the same facilitator 'pairs' should be available to take at least one, if not both, sessions at each level. Indeed, this has been achieved by several facilitator 'pairs', and their success has been recognised in the student evaluations, expressed in free text comments such as 'they knew each, other making the atmosphere relaxed'; 'they were part of the group'.

The joint learning and teaching ideal does place extremely heavy demands on the availability of facilitators, and pairing for the majority is not always possible. It is often the case that the facilitators do not meet until five minutes before a session begins. However, in some instances the pair may have taken a shared ethics session before and therefore are able to establish a rapport more readily. Conversely, it may be the case that the pair are meeting for the first time and find it difficult to present a unified front. This is expressed in student comments such as 'the ice should be broken earlier' and, from the same cohort, 'air of tension, one late and presumed authority . . . not a good start for introducing teaching between nurses and doctors'.

It is acknowledged that the majority of facilitators have chosen to teach on these ethics courses, but problems arise simply because of other clinical, managerial and educational commitments.

Action
Shared ethics facilitator teams have been formed in an attempt to ameliorate the situation. This allows a degree of flexibility for all involved, and also leads to a more secure timetable pattern.

Issue 4. Student knowledge base

This issue concerns the matching of student knowledge. The challenge to find a suitable point in the respective student programmes where each cohort has a similar, compatible knowledge base of ethics and clinical experience has been difficult. Although both curricula contain the topic of ethics, each has a different point and time where this subject is delivered and the hours allocated vary considerably.

Despite these problems it is evident that the students strongly favour the experience of meeting together to discuss ethical issues.

It is encouraging to hear and read the same positive comments year after year. 'It gives an insight as to how other professionals think on the field of ethics'; 'both medical and nursing students saw each others points of view'; 'enjoyed the session and found it useful'; 'best ethics session yet'; 'enjoyed joint participation'; 'the session was very good, having different views and opinions'; 'well presented, well run'; 'held everyone's attention'; 'good to have multi-professional approach'.

Action
The co-ordinators and steering group continue to monitor and liaise with programme leaders within both schools to evaluate the impact of curricular changes on the shared teaching venture.

Issue 5. Staff development

Staff development in the form of facilitator workshops was identified as important to the shared teaching concept. Various efforts have been made to establish regular workshops. To date only three have been successfully effected. These sessions afforded the facilitators the opportunity to explore and debate the relevant ethical issues inherent within the scenarios. However, the logistics of bringing together two groups of healthcare professionals, both with differing commitments, has been at times insurmountable.

Action
In an attempt to improve attendance at these events, the timing and venues have been varied.

Conclusion to reality

The honesty proffered within this section will hopefully assist those planning to initiate inter-professional and multi-professional teaching for healthcare professionals. There are times when one has to be cautious and other times when one has to move quickly, firmly, with courage and determination. Yes, there are still problems to overcome however as the evaluation results show the experience is worthy of the endeavours.

Evaluation

Within any course of study it is necessary to measure the quality of the teaching strategy used and assess if those taking part have valued the experience (Pelligrino, 1989). Therefore, evaluations of the shared teaching in ethics were effected to achieve this standard (see Appendices 6.1–6.3). The results of the evaluations have played a significant role in moulding and improving the three levels. At the same time, the co-ordinators have been conscious of not subjecting the students and facilitators to 'evaluation over kill'.

Conclusion

In 1993 when the junior level was initiated it was not fully appreciated how it would evolve. The evaluations undertaken provided direction and assisted the shape of future developments. However, whilst it can be tempting to be charmed into a static position with the positive results of innovation it is also necessary to recognise and address the problems and challenges which remain. In essence, the concept of the idea into reality has been a complex a long process.

The process of moving forward required analysis of the experiences of both the students and the facilitators who participated in all the sessions. This required reflection and sensitivity to the expressions and opinions of all involved. Despite evidence that the students and facilitators valued the sessions so far, there is no research evidence to support the view that these endeavours will produce benefit to the consumers within the healthcare settings. Research, although at an embryonic stage, is presently addressing this issue.

The progress to date has required vision, determination, courage, considerable goodwill and support from all participants. However, what has been clearly recognised is the importance of these sessions and the necessity to continue to meet the challenges as they occur. Indeed, if we can grasp the interest of the students and assist then to identify the relevance and importance of the very reasons and nature of shared teaching in ethics, then the future looks bright.

References

Casto, R M and Julie, M C (1994) *Interprofessional Care and Collaborative Practice*. Pacific Grove, CA, USA Brooks Cole Publishing.

Edward, C and Preece, P E (1999) Shared Teaching in Health Care Ethics Report on the Beginning of an Idea, *Nursing Ethics*, **6**(4), 229–307.

Ekeli, B-V (1996) *Multiprofessional Learning in Health Care Education in Tromso*, paper presented at 22nd World Congress of Medical Technology, Oslo, Norway.

Forbes, E J and Fitzsimons, V (1993) Education: The Key for Holistic Interdisciplinary Collaboration, *Holistic Nursing Practice*, **7**(4), 1–10.

Holm, S (1997) *Ethical Problems in Clinical Practice: The Ethical Reasoning of Health Care Professionals*. Manchester: Manchester University Press.

Krawczyk, R and Kudzma, E (1978) Ethics: A Matter of Moral Development, *Nursing Outlook*, April, **26**, 254–7.

McKiel, R E, Lockyer, J and Pechiulis, D D (1998) A Model of Continuing Education for Conjoint Practice, *The Journal of Continuing Education in Nursing*, **19**(2), 65–7.

Mitchell, K R, Lovat, T J and Mysler, C M (1992) *Medical Education*, **26**, 290–300.

Pelligrino, E D (1989) Teaching Medical Ethics: Some Persistent Questions and Some Responses, *Academic Medicine*, December.

Peter, E and Gallop, R (1994) The Ethics of Care: A Comparison of Nursing and Medical Students, *Image: Journal of Nursing Scholarship*, **26**(1), 47–51.

Platt, L J, Casto, R M and Julie, M C (1994) *Interprofessional Care and Collaborative Practice*, Ch. 1, Why Bother With Teams?: An Overview.

Rodgers, J and Fry, N (1994) Collaboration Among Health Professionals, *Nursing Standard*, **9**(6), 25–6.

Seedhouse, D (1988) *Ethics: the Heart of Caring* (reprinted 1993). Chichster John Wiley and Sons.

Self, D J, Wolinsky, F D and Baldwin de, W C (1989) The Effect of Teaching Medical Ethics on Medical Students' Moral Reasoning, *Academic Medicine*, December, 755–9.

Soothill, K, Mackay, L and Webb, C (1994) *Inter professional Relationships in Health care*, Second Edition. Chapter 1 Troubled Times: the context of inter professional collaboration. London: Edward Arnold.

de Tournay, R (1994) In Larsan, E L, DeBasio, N O, Mundinger, M O, Shoemaker J K (1995) *Interdisciplinary Education and Practice*, American Association of Colleges of Nursing Position Statement.

Vitz, P C (1990) The Use of Stories in Moral Development: New Psychological Reasons for an Old Education Method, *American Psychologist*, **45**(6), 709–20.

Wall, A (1993) *Ethics and The Health Service Manager*, London, King Edwards Fund.

WHO (World Health Organisation) (1988) *Learning Together to Work Together for Health*. Report of WHO Study Group on Multipro-fessional Education of Health Personnel: The Team Approach, WHO Technical Report series 769, Geneva: WHO.

Ytrehus, I (1993) Multiprofessional Education in Health Services in Tromso Norway, paper presented at conference 'Towards Quality in Multiprofessional Education and Work', European Network for Development of Multiprofessional Education in Health Sciences (EMPE), Krakow, Poland.

Appendix Students' evaluations of the sessions

Junior level

To evaluate this stage of shared teaching the students were invited to complete a questionnaire at the conclusion of the session. Comments collated are as follows.

'Did the facilitators in your group work in harmony?'

Responses
- Both facilitators joined in bringing in their personal experience which I found useful.
- Well organised.
- Yes, they worked in harmony and allowed the group to develop discussion.
- Good to have both medical and nursing represented.
- Doctors tried to dominate the session and talked too much.
- I do not think that they communicated well together ... there seemed to be a lot of tension and answers coming from one end and not the other.

Was the classroom environment suitable for the session?

Responses
- The chairs were in a circle and this was comfortable for discussion.
- By sitting in a circle it enables everybody to see each other and maximise contribution.

- Classroom was lovely...do not have anything like it in the medical school.
- Too big.

Please write down any negative or positive aspects of the session

Responses
- Everyone could express their own opinion although it was a long session.
- Learned a lot form other disciplines.
- It gave you insight as to how other professionals think of ethics.
- Some people talked all the time.
- Felt that medical students looked at the physical aspects rather than the ethical issues.
- Do not like nurses.
- Enjoyed getting different points of view from the nursing students.
- Half of the group did not turn up ...enjoyed session and gained a lot of vital information.
- Divide between medical and nursing students.
- Some scenarios short on information...could have done with some definitive legal issues.
- Its a Friday afternoon.
- Too much ethics this week.

The facilitators were invited to comment on their experience of the shared teaching. Comments collated are as follows.

Please state any negative or positive points about the session

Responses
- Useful to see medical and nursing students together.
- I thought that the students interacted very well.
- Significant number of non-attendance...excellent session with those who attended.
- Extremely enjoyable session.
- Co-facilitator late in arriving.
- Too many scenarios and some did not provoke immediate response and the outcomes were similar.
- Co-facilitator wanted to take over the session.

- Problem with rooms...changed at the last moment...area was noisy.
- The facilitator I was with talked too much and appeared to be more interested in the legal aspect of the case.

Intermediate level

To evaluate this stage of shared teaching the students were invited to complete a questionnaire at the conclusion of the session. Comments collated are as follows.

Please state any negative or positive aspects of the course

Responses
- Liked the group work and we were left alone with the facilitators only briefly monitoring the situation.
- Treated like adults.
- Would have been better if there had been more nursing students in our group.
- Bit nervous to begin with but it was really good.
- Medics very little knowledge about ethics.
- Session was too long.
- Balance of nurse to medics was uneven.
- Interesting scenarios.
- Not really told what the session was about beforehand.
- Some people were not interested.
- Ice breaker was embarrassing.
- Enjoyed mixing with nursing students.

As before the facilitators were invited to comment on the shared teaching experience. Comments collated are as follows

Please state any negative or positive aspects of the course

Responses
- Nurses good at ethics, medical students at law.
- Excellent session.
- Students worked well together.
- Poor attendance.
- Student package excellent.
- Nurses said very little.

- Nurses very vocal.
- More variation in topics for discussion, e.g. genetic engineering and radical, surgery.
- More time, e.g. all day.

Senior level

In May 1998 one session only took place: 'Resuscitation . . . Who decides?' The free text comments of the evaluation are as follows

Responses
- The session was very good.
- Session was too short.
- The session was different and more interesting than a normal lecture on such a controversial topic.
- It was well organised.
- Felt that the issues were not answered in full detail, just skirted around.
- Discussion occurred mostly in the panel.
- Boring-required much more interaction between us and the lecturers/speakers and also each other.
- Nice chance to interact with people out of our class, seniors other health workers.
- Far too long and not very interesting.

At the time of writing the planned session on 'The rights and wrongs of end of life issues' has yet to be delivered.

7

Evaluation of an Inter-professional Training Ward: Pilot Phase

Della Freeth and Scott Reeves

Introduction

This chapter describes, from the evaluators' perspective, the development and pilot phase of an Inter-professional training ward placement for medical, nursing, occupational therapy and physiotherapy students. The four-week training ward pilot, which ran from February to March 1999 within Barts and The London NHS Trust, was the first such educational venture in the UK. A multi-method evaluation of the pilot phase was undertaken by the authors, who continue to be involved with the training ward's development and evaluation.

The St Bartholomew School of Nursing and Midwifery, City University and the St Bartholomew and The Royal London School of Medicine and Dentistry, Queen Mary and Westfield College, London University (QMW) have a long history of commitment to collaboration in the development of inter-professional education (Studdy *et al.*, 1994; Dacre and Nicol, 1996; Freeth and Nicol, 1998; Reeves and Pryce, 1998). This is unusual between medical and nursing schools in England. The collaboration between these two schools is also remarkable, first, in having survived the schools' incorporations into different universities, and second, in focusing on pre-registration education which generally poses greater logistical challenges than post-registration education.

The inter-professional training ward, London

In 1996 the then Deans of School at City and QMW, with two educational development specialists, visited Linköping in Sweden, where the first inter-professional training ward had been established (Sandén and Wahlström, 1996; Wahlström and Sandén, 1998). Following this, a project steering group was established to plan a London-based training ward that would include students of medicine, nursing, occupational therapy and physiotherapy. The training ward model pioneered in Sweden was to be adapted in the light of the Swedish experience and evaluation, and also to meet the needs and aspirations of service providers, educators and students in Inner London – a very different social context to Linköping.

Membership of the steering committee was drawn from the originating schools at City and QMW, Barts and the London NHS Trust (where the ward was to be located), Tower Hamlets Health Care Trust (who would provide supervision for the occupational therapy students), the School of Occupational Therapy at QMW, and the Department of Physiotherapy at the University of East London. Thus, the training ward project required collaboration from two NHS trusts and four schools in three universities. It is not surprising, therefore, that the training ward pilot had a gestation period of 18 months, during which there were several changes of personnel in the planning team.

The literature on inter-professional collaboration indicates that inter-professional initiatives require more planning time than uni-professional initiatives and also are particularly vulnerable when key staff change (see e.g. Carpenter, 1995). Simply mounting the training ward pilot should be regarded as a significant achievement to be celebrated. It is, therefore, worthy of further celebration that the pilot was judged to be successful and that the partner institutions are, at the time of writing, working towards establishing an inter-professional training ward placement as an integral part of senior students' educational programmes. The training ward used for the pilot project is due to recommence on a continuing basis later this year.

The training ward occupied a 12-bedded section of a 27-bed orthopaedic and rheumatology ward. In the four week pilot period two cohorts of three inter-professional student teams completed a two-week placement. Each team comprised two medical students, two nursing students and one occupational therapy (OT) student, all in their final year of study, in addition to one second year physiotherapy (PT) student. Students' learning aims for the training ward centred around promoting teamwork within a real clinical setting, developing their own professional roles and gaining an insight into other professional roles. Under the supervision of practitioners from each of the disciplines, but particularly a senior nurse facilitator who worked the same shifts (morning or afternoon) as her team throughout the pilot, the students planned and delivered care to patients. To update one another, student teams undertook inter-professional handovers at the beginning and end of their shifts. All students undertook a range of duties: duties that were specific to their profession and also duties that were designed to encourage inter-professional teamwork.

Patients were selected for participation in the training ward on the basis of their clinical needs, particularly a need for input from each of the participating professions. They gave special informed consent to receive their care on the training ward.

The educational philosophy selected for the training ward was problem-based learning (PBL). In addition to their on-ward patient care, after each morning shift students attended reflective sessions where they could discuss their ward experiences and develop/review their PBL learning objectives. These sessions were facilitated by tutors from one of the three participating schools or one of the trust-based, profession-specific facilitators. The practitioners who acted as team facilitators or profession-specific facilitators were offered training, led by school-based facilitators, relating to the theory and implementation of PBL. Most of the relevant staff were able to attend this, and there was a certain amount of informal training between colleagues when the formal sessions had been missed.

Evaluation

The evaluation was formative in orientation. There were many stakeholders from different disciplines to satisfy, and information on both processes and outcomes was required. Consequently, a multi-method approach was adopted with data collection before, during and after the training ward pilot.

The evaluators began attending steering group meetings approximately one year before the pilot ran. From this point, their analysis of the literature and interpretation of observations they made during a short visit to the Swedish training ward in October 1998 may be considered to have had some influence on the planning process. Thus the researcher stance was closer to action research than detached observer with findings and interpretations being fed back to the training ward steering group throughout the evaluation.

Data collection included: observations at meetings; handovers; reflection sessions and during, training; observations; on the ward; individual and focus-group interviews with staff and students which were tape recorded and transcribed; questionnaires completed by students and patients; and reflective journals offered by some facilitators.

Discussion of evaluation findings

Virtually everyone who contributed to the evaluation was, on balance, positive about the achievements and opportunities of the training ward pilot. No one suggested that the training ward should not run again and no one suggested wholesale revision of the model. Patients, students and staff were keen to see the training ward develop and thrive. Collectively, they made a large number of suggestions for the improvement and development of the ward. These have been interpreted as helpful, constructive criticism, not a litany of complaint.

In the evaluation report (Freeth and Reeves, 1999) findings were presented thematically under ten major headings, with some being further elaborated with sub-themes. The major themes drew together the perspectives of patients, students and staff, with each theme drawing upon both qualitative and quantitative data relating to each of the three phases of data collection: before, during and after the training ward pilot. The themes that are described overlap, but are useful to structure and illuminate the multi-faceted nature of the training ward experience. In order to present a detailed but concise account of our findings we focus upon six of the major themes. These are outlined below.

1. Real life

Staff and students very much valued the training ward place-ment as providing an experience that was closer to 'real life' than normal student placements. At times this was experienced as overwhelming, but students generally responded well to being asked to take greater responsibility for planning patient care and their own work priorities:

> I think they are going to be better prepared to make decisions and hopefully it is going to help them get from student status to [*profession*] status. (p-facilitator – see Glossary, p. xx)

> I think it is great to be thrown in at the deep end because that is what will happen...it [provides] a much more realistic picture. (n-facilitator – see Glossary, p. xx)

Like the facilitators, students considered the 'real-life' experience of planning and delivering care for patients as one of the most beneficial aspects of their ward placement. They particularly val-ued the increased levels of responsibility and autonomy they had on the ward: an experience which allowed a better opportunity for them to 'think through' (PT student) and decide how they could best care for patients. The training ward placement was widely regarded as offering a striking contrast to conventional clinical placements, where supervisors tended to lead in patient care. Students also felt that the training ward provided them with a good insight into the practical issues of managing the pressures of a clinical workload:

> Even when everyone is on the phone and that's a hassle, it teaches you what to expect in the future (m-student)

> I feel I got a lot of confidence and responsibility which really prepared me for when I qualify, so that has been a valuable part of it (n-student)

In many respects the value students and facilitators placed on the 'real-life' aspect of the ward is not surprising since adult learners are life centred and problem based (Knowes, 1990; Rogers, 1969).

Similarly, it has been reported that inter-professional education is enhanced for participants when it is directly linked to their current or future clinical practice (e.g. Parsell *et al.*, 1998; Miller *et al.*, 1999). For Thomas (1995:212) the quality of inter-professional education is maximised when there is 'fidelity between educational programmes and the real world'. However, as these findings also suggest, care is needed to ensure that this 'real-life' experience is not too overwhelming, especially for inexperienced learners.

2. Learning and teaching

The learning and teaching theme has five sub-themes: facilitation; student support; off-ward learning; studying the relevant theory; student learning objectives; and the two-week placement. In addition, this theme is closely related to the third theme, the problem-based approach.

Facilitation
Students received two types of facilitation during their placement: profession-specific facilitation from their own professional supervisors and also team facilitation from nurse-facilitators.

Profession-specific facilitation varied between professions in approach and frequency, and varying degrees of satisfaction were expressed. The profession-specific facilitators added this role to their existing workloads for the period of the pilot. Many felt that they could not continue with this arrangement over the long term.

Attached to each student team was a nurse facilitator who provided students with team-orientated facilitation throughout their shifts and also acted as a resource for all members of the student team. During the pilot each facilitator was responsible for two teams, one team in the first two weeks and another team in the remaining two weeks. The nurse facilitators found their team facilitation duties very demanding and expressed a desire for ongoing support with the implementation of PBL. Concerns were expressed that, if the training ward is to run on a continuous basis, the potential for burnout among these staff should be considered.

Nurse facilitators each developed their own style over the course of the pilot. These different styles were observed to influence team functioning and are reflected in the following extracts.

> She did leave us to our own devices (n-student – see Glossary, p. xx)
>
> We allowed [*the nurse facilitator*] to co-ordinate us. (PT student)
>
> [*The nurse facilitator*] viewed it as a team exercise and made us feel accountable as members of the team. (PT student)

However, each of the nurse-facilitators modified her style during the training ward pilot as she grew into the role.

> For the first two weeks my team was up and down like a see-saw, because to start with we started one [*facilitation*] pattern and then you'd find it is not working ... and then you would change ... because it is new you have to find your own feet, because you are not sure what you are doing. (n-facilitator)

The nurse-facilitators also varied in the extent to which they participated in the team's ward work. Where this participation was high it reduced stress and friction by making it easier for the team to complete their work on time but did not necessarily encourage all members of the team to participate fully in the team's work.

> We just decided, right you do your job, I'll do mine ... we run pretty much as a normal ward would. (n-student)

The role of facilitator within interprofessional education is regarded as critical in shaping the overall experience for learners (e.g. Funnell, 1995; Parsell *et al.*, 1998). It is argued that in order to make a positive impact in this type of learning, facilitators need to pay attention to both the formation and the maintenance of the learner team. In doing so, it is argued that the opportunities for enhancing collaboration can be emphasised (e.g. Casto, 1994; Headrick *et al.*, 1998). The facilitation of inter-professional teams on the ward requires more development and research. At present, it would appear that a good approach would emphasise team functioning and accountability, and would offer a reasonably high level of support and direction during the first one or two shifts, such support rapidly tailing off thereafter.

Student support

Students wanted more support and direction in the early part of their placement concerning how they 'manage' the training ward. This is closely linked with the fifth theme, preparation. Some students also expressed a desire for feedback from facilitators concerning their individual and team performances during the training ward placement:

> Maybe we could have some more support when we started and were trying to find our feet. (n-student)

> Everyone's got their profession-specific role but on this particular project, for two weeks, we are working on this together. How we do it [*work together*] was never gone into in depth. (n-student)

The anxieties expressed by the students on the ward were not unexpected. Learners in unfamiliar milieu do experience a temporary reduction in self-confidence and increased anxiety (Bloomfield, 1997). Learners therefore seek greater contact with their tutors and ask for the learning experience to be structured for them. They need time to 'suss out' the demands of the new learning environment (Morgan, 1993). Once this process is completed, learners' confidence and competencies, which they have developed in the process of successful learning in a variety of milieu, return and are enhanced by the success in the most recent milieu. Tutors receiving students in unfamiliar learning environments should be aware of that an initial desire for increased dependency is normal, predictable and temporary. With the benefit of this insight, tutors can more effectively plan and manage students' successful adaptation to the unfamiliar learning milieu.

Off-ward learning

Two types of off-ward learning session were facilitated by staff: planned team reflection sessions after each morning shift, and patient review sessions in the early part of each team's placement, instigated by the medical facilitators. The patient review sessions were considered useful in overcoming students' initial problems with patient management, provided that each professional group was able to contribute fully.

Team reflection sessions, facilitated by staff from three of the participating schools, and also attended by the nurse-facilitators, were generally viewed as a positive element of the training ward experience. They embraced a variety of student concerns about the ward, including:

- managing the ward workload effectively
- difficulties around the participation in team duties

- concern about the initial lack of facilitator support on the ward
- student uncertainty about what the training ward would entail
- coping with the stresses of weekday morning shifts
- lack of time and opportunity for an insight into other students' professional roles
- concern that the ward disrupted students' final year examination preparation.

Although it was originally planned to use these sessions for generating and reviewing student learning objectives, 11 reflection sessions were observed and this occurred only once. Facilitators experienced some uncertainty over the required facilitation of team reflection sessions. One tutor explained that this was due to an intellectual distinction between facilitating PBL and facilitating reflection.

> I found it hard to know how much I could intervene or suggest things. If it is PBL I am not allowed to do much. If it's reflection I can lead them and try to help them make sense of practice and see what they are learning ... my feeling is that we should forget the PBL bit and call it reflection on what they are learning. (p-facilitator)

The problems associated with the inconsistent use of these sessions needs further attention. Clearly, future staff development work with facilitators could be devoted to strengthening this aspect of the training ward.

The value of reflection within inter-professional education is stressed in the inter-professional education literature (e.g. Howkins and Allison 1997; Parsell *et al.*, 1998). Indeed, for Pietroni (1991) the use of reflection is a necessary component in encouraging learners to move from a sole focus on their own profession to developing an awareness of the contribution of other professions in patient care.

Student learning objectives

Students were expected to meet around ten profession-specific and also 19 'generic' team-oriented learning objectives during their two-week ward placement. This was found to be too many to be successfully completed within this relatively short time span. In addition, there was some tension between profession-specific development and teamwork development.

> Everybody is looking to achieve their own [*profession-specific*] object-
> ives and still work together and that is hard (n-facilitator).

This finding has resonance with work by Dienst and Byl (1981)
who encountered a similar tension between students achieving both
profession-specific learning and team-based learning objectives
in their inter-professional education course for medical, nursing,
pharmacy and physiotherapy students. These authors note that
for many students team-based learning was not seen to be as
important as their profession-specific learning. Indeed, recently
published work from the Linköping ward also found that the
Swedish students also encountered tension between developing
both their profession-specific objectives and their teamwork objectives (Fallsberg and Wijma, 1999). Early feedback from the evaluators to the steering group has resulted in a commitment to
focus the ward on just four objectives in future, emphasising
teamwork.

The two-week placement
The two week placement was felt by many to be too short: teams
were just beginning to function effectively when the placement
ended.

> I think about three weeks because you have got your first week to
> establish yourself, your second week to really start to get to know
> everything and your last week which would be like, 'I've got it, I'm
> doing this right'. (n-student)

This has resonance with the literature on team formation and
functioning (e.g. McGrath, 1990; Jaques 1984). This literature
indicates that teams need time to evolve and develop, with each
team passing through a number of complex 'phases' from beginning to the end of their 'lifespan'. McGrath (1990) stresses that
time is important in teams and suggests that teams who have
a short lifespan tend to 'rush' through their development which
often produces poorer-quality inter-team communication and team
member support. For Jacques (1984) improved group cohesion
and communication requires a sense of trust and openness which
takes time to develop between group members. Early feedback of
this finding has resulted in the steering group trying to extend
placements to three weeks in the next phase.

3. The problem-based approach

The training ward was designed to provide students with a real-life clinical experience in which students, with help of their facilitators, employed a PBL approach to resolving the numerous problems of planning and delivering patient care. However, both students and facilitators encountered a variety of difficulties with PBL on the ward. Staff in particular were mainly concerned with how much help they were 'allowed' to give students, resulting in facilitators adopting differing approaches to PBL.

> A student came to me and said 'the number on the name band is different to the number on the drug chart'. And I said to her what would she do and she said, 'I'll check it'. And I said, 'Right, where would you check it?' And she stood there for about five minutes and didn't know and I said, 'Ok, check the medical notes'. And [a senior colleague] said to me, 'You are not supposed to be telling them where to find it, they are supposed to be finding it themselves.'... [The student] identified the problem, she identified what she needed to do, but didn't know how to do it and I think she needed that input. (n-facilitator)

Some students felt the training ward experience had not employed PBL because they were too busy dealing with the practicalities of managing patient care to be aware of or give time to PBL. Others felt that the stress on PBL was a red herring in that it amounted to unfamiliar jargon for a familiar process.

> We haven't done PBL... we were so busy just keeping on top of daily ward business. (OT student)

> We don't call this PBL, we call this patient management. (m-student – see Glossary)

Although PBL is widely employed within inter-professional education (e.g. Hughes and Lucas, 1997; Snadden and Bain, 1998) most initiatives use this educational approach with small groups in classroom settings where there is time for debate and discussion. As found during the pilot, such an approach can be more problemat-based within the real-world demands of the clinical environment.

In addition, it has been known for some time that attempting to adopt a deep approach to learning, without adequate prior knowledge, when time is short, can be associated with failure (Ent-wistle, 1987). Perhaps it was overoptimistic to attempt to implement PBL in a time-constrained situation with several facilitators who were new to PBL and, of necessity, with all facilitators being unfamiliar with the realities of the inter-professional training ward placement. Lack of prior knowledge and experience will, of course, be dimin-ishing problems if the training ward runs on a continued basis.

Overall, students and facilitators recognised that a PBL approach had potential to improve learning from the training ward place-ment. Nevertheless, they felt more time was needed, away from the ward, to be able to focus upon each professional group's con-tribution to patient care.

4. Team duties

In order to provide students with opportunities which would allow them to work closely together on the ward, students undertook shared 'team' duties such as making beds or washing patients. Team duties were intended to allow students to develop communi-cation and teamworking skills, which could ultimately enhance their inter-professional relationships. In addition, involvement in these team duties was seen as helping students develop a better understanding of one another's roles and pressures in the deliv-ery of care. Staff also considered there was scope for team duties to contribute to profession-specific knowledge and development. For example, occupational therapy and physiotherapy students could assess patients during a transfer from bed to commode. However, as these duties essentially revolved around tasks gen-erally perceived as nurse-orientated work, it was anticipated that problems could be encountered with non-nursing students.

Data collected during and after the pilot confirmed that non-nursing students saw team duties as nursing duties, although the nursing students disagreed. They felt that many of the team duties would normally have been undertaken by a health care assistant and that interpreting team duties as nursing duties rep-resented a distorted view of the nature of nursing practice.

[*The other students think*] nursing care is giving someone their dinner or giving them a bowl of water or washing people. (n-student)

For some, the perceived nursing orientation produced a reluctance to participate in team duties and some teams faced significant interpersonal difficulties related to this issue.

For some facilitators, student participation in team duties was regarded as an unrealistic version of interprofessional teamwork.

> The students are all expected to work as a team and muck in and help each other. That is not how teams work in reality. (p-facilitator)

Furthermore, medical students, willing or otherwise, found it difficult to participate fully in team duties since most were undertaken in the mornings. This clashed with consultant ward rounds that were greater in number than planned (because an unexpectedly large number of consultants had patients on the training ward) and unpredictable in timing.

Students from all professions felt that the emphasis on team duties, and the particular tasks designated as team duties, restricted their ability to gain an accurate insight into the roles and expertise of the four professions involved. This links with the sub-theme (above) of student learning objectives. It was felt that sharing tasks normally associated with one profession was problematic and not necessarily the best vehicle for developing understanding of each other's roles.

> We can help them [*nursing students*], but they can't really help us with presenting and the writing up of notes. (m-student)

> The aim [*of the training ward*] is to understand each other's job, not be able to do it. (p-facilitator)

Student participation in team duties presents a number of problems for the training ward. The logistic problems preventing some students taking place in this aspect of the ward could easily be resolved in a future reorganisation of the ward. However, the problem of role sharing which the team duties demand is a more sensitive difficulty to overcome. As indicated, student participation in team duties resulted in friction as they encountered problems over role overlap.

When one considers the teamwork literature such problems are not surprising. In considering what factors make up an 'effective' team, one discovers that clearly defined team roles are crucial. Thus role overlap undermines the team's effectiveness in working together (e.g. West, 1997; Elywin *et al* 1998). Indeed, this issue is often commonly cited in the inter-professional education literature as students are generally found to be protective of their own professional 'turf' and resist perceived attempts to undermine their professional role (e.g. Itano *et al.*, 1991, Pirrie *et al.*, 1998).

In attempting to resolve the problems around team duties, the steering group are currently considering 'role shadowing' as a more productive way to learn about roles and their pressures.

5. Training ward patients

During the planning of the training ward pilot the majority of facilitators and ward staff anticipated advantages for patients on the ward.

> I think they [*training ward patients*] will probably get better care than the other patients... because they [*the students*] have got more time to sit with them, ask different things and discover problems that on a general ward would be missed. (p-facilitator)

Nevertheless, there were a concerns around patient involvement in the training ward. These centred on four aspects:

1. It was felt that 'suitable' training ward patients would need to be at a 'fairly low risk of being really ill' (p-facilitator) and to require input from all the student groups.
2. Concern was expressed that patients should give special consent that demonstrated awareness of the students' contribution to their care.
3. It was felt that patients' relatives may be reluctant for them to participate in the training ward.
4. Staff felt that procedures needed to be in place to ensure the rapid transfer of any training ward patient who became very unwell.

All these issues were addressed before the pilot began. Indeed, post-training ward interviews revealed that initial expectations around the training ward patients receiving more attention than patients elsewhere were met. Staff and students considered the mix of patients was 'about right' (p-facilitator) for the student teams. It was felt that students, on the whole, managed these patients in a proficient manner. Similarly, staff and students felt that 12 patients was a suitable number for this type of student experience, although one facilitator felt strongly that the number of patients be reduced to ten in order to reduce the student workload. It was acknowledged that students received some conflicting demands and advice from different medical teams.

Obtaining special patient consent was regarded as problematic for staff during the pilot period. Ethical approval for the pilot was conditional upon obtaining daily verbal consent from patients to remain on the training ward, in addition to initial written consent. For the staff responsible this duty was a time-consuming burden. It was felt that more streamlined processes needed to be developed for the ongoing project.

Patients were positive about their care on the training ward. Having six students and a nurse facilitator available to meet their needs resulted in more 'staff' – patient contact and communication than these patients had experienced elsewhere in the hospital. This was felt to be advantageous, apart from raised levels of noise that could disturb the most ill. Patients reported that team efficiency improved during the two-week placement.

> As the week has gone by they [*the students*] have got better. (patient)
>
> [*The students*] are excellent. I can't fault them. One hundred per cent service. (patient)
>
> More staff [*i.e. students*], more individual attention and information. (patient)

When compared to similar patients in adjacent clinical areas, training ward patients expressed more satisfaction with their care, particularly in relation to: students/staff listening; answering patient questions; providing information to patients; and meeting patient needs. Training ward patients' responses revealed a perception that students tended to inform one another about individual patient care more than staff on conventional wards.

These findings are helpful in beginning to establish the impact of this type of inter-professional education on patient care. Indeed, with the increasing need to establish a firm evidence base for practice (e.g. Department of Health, 1998), this focus on patient care is highly appropriate. This is especially the case when one considers the current lack of evidence for the effects of inter-professional education on patient care. Despite some useful evidence indicating the potential benefits on learners (e.g. Hughes and Lucas, 1997; Parsell *et al.*, 1998), little is known in relation to its effects on patients (Zwarenstein *et al.*, 1999).

To strengthen this aspect of future evaluations it is hoped to obtain hospital audit data on length of stay, readmission rates, etc. This will allow the evaluators to begin to assess, more objectively, the impact of inter-professional education on the training ward for patient care.

Impact of the training ward on service delivery

Supervising practitioners ensured that the care delivered to patients was safe and appropriate. One patient experienced an adverse reaction during the pilot and this tested the medical supervision in particular, but was resolved safely. A small number of supervisors had reservations about teams' ability to progress care in a timely manner, especially during the first week of each placement. Trust staff felt that patients' stay on the training ward was slightly longer than it would normally have been, but we were told that the situation was no worse than when the pre-registration house officers rotate. The cost of a marginally increased length of stay may have been more than offset by savings from not allocating a health care assistant to the training ward. At the time of writing, it has not been possible to triangulate this finding with audit data, since anonymised audit data is not yet available to the evaluators.

It was reported that placing the less complicated patients in the training ward resulted in a heavier patient workload for adjacent clinical areas. The impact of this burden was felt to have been exacerbated because three of the directorate's more experienced nurses were occupied in the training ward as nurse facilitators. However, there was disagreement over whether this was a real problem for the delivery of the service or an issue of reduced staff morale and slight inconvenience among those not chosen to participate in the training ward pilot.

Staff across the directorate felt the training ward would increase the prestige of the directorate and the trust, and that this might help with the recruitment and retention of staff.

> I think the thing is it will encourage and increase recruitment because people will want to work on a ward that is new and the first in the country. (ward staff)

However, an area of concern emerged. Staff felt that establishing the training ward would essentially split the larger ward into 'two separate little wards' (ward staff), each with their own identity. For these staff there was a feeling that the training ward could 'cause quite a division' (ward staff) between the two ward areas. In particular, it was considered that most of the attention and activity would be focused on the training ward, leaving staff in 'normal' ward area feeling 'just a little elbowed out' (ward staff).

Facilitators viewed the prospect of working on the training ward positively. They were enthusiastic about contributing to the UK's first training ward, and emphasised that the experience would contribute to their personal, professional and academic development.

> It is a chance for me to use my academic knowledge and put that into practice. (n-facilitator)

In addition, facilitators regarded the ward as an opportunity to deepen their own understanding of other professional roles.

> I don't know what the physiotherapist's role is entirely. (p-facilitator)

Although facilitators enjoyed their work with the students on the training ward, they had underestimated the amount of input they would be required to make. In addition to the demands of the training ward, the nurse facilitators were called upon to help the qualified nursing staff in adjacent clinical areas.

> [I was] called upon to deal with issues outside the training ward, colleagues looking for support. (n-facilitator)

It was felt that clinical staff should rotate in and out of training ward facilitator posts. This would allow all interested staff to become more involved in the training ward and also protect facilitators from occupational 'burn-out'.

To overcome these initial difficulties (e.g. facilitator burn-out) and in order to establish the training ward as a successful inter-professional initiative, it is vital that the ward receives ongoing institutional support. Casto (1994) and Pirrie *et al.*, (1998) consider that it is necessary to ensure funding, staff and resources can be all made available in order to secure the long-term running of this type of innovative professional education.

Conclusions

Hawthorne effect

It is known that being the focus of managerial and research attention may generate improvements in morale and output that are not sustained in the long run, the 'Hawthorne effect'. It is not possible to be certain whether, or to what extent, this effect altered the outcomes of the training ward pilot and its evaluation. However, it is possible that any losses occurring from a diminishing Hawthorne effect may be more than offset by improvements in the continuing project arising from learning from the pilot.

Strengths of the training ward pilot

- The training ward initiative is unique in the UK. Early national and international dissemination of the evaluation has sparked a great deal of interest. The initiative seems certain to raise the profile of the two participating NHS trusts and four participating schools.
- Over a prolonged period, the training ward benefited from facilitative support and commitment from trust and university staff at all levels. This was pivotal to the successful running of the pilot.
- The 'real-life' clinical experience with which the training ward provided students was the most highly valued aspect of the ward placement.

- By being provided with more autonomy to make clinical decisions, students developed confidence and obtained a beneficial insight into their future professional practice. Students did not feel they usually received this kind of insight with their traditional clinical placements.
- Students valued the input they received from the interprofessional the patient review sessions.
- In addition, students highly regarded their team reflection sessions, where they could discuss and reflect upon their ward-based work.
- Patients were very satisfied with the care and attention they received.
- It was generally considered that 12 patients was an appropriate number for students to manage. It was felt that students, on the whole, coped well with the mix of patients during the ward placement. All patient cases allowed students from the four professional groups some input.
- The training ward pilot provided an innovative educational experience for students and a career development opportunity for associated staff.

Future development

The training ward pilot ran successfully. However, to overcome the teething problems and preserve the pilot's strengths, the following recommendations are made.

- To overcome the identified problems connected with students' ability to manage the 'real-life' demands placed on them, and also to provide them with a less dramatic shift from a traditional form of learning to a more autonomous one on the training ward, more preparation and initial support could be given to assist students with this transition.
- Particular attention should be paid to the role of facilitator: the number and experience of staff selected for this role, their initial training and ongoing support, and arrangements for rotation in and out of this role.
- Due to their ward-based workload, students found it was difficult to obtain a substantial insight into professional roles of

the medical, OT and PT students. They may also have gained a distorted impression of the nursing role, focused on a narrow range of tasks. As this is an essential feature of the inter-professional ward experience, students should be encouraged to work-shadow one another. Indeed, time should be allocated for this.

- The PBL approach used in the training ward generated a good deal of confusion for both facilitators and students. It may be worth reconsidering the use of PBL in the next phase of the training ward. To reduce this confusion, especially the difficulties facilitators encountered with knowing how much direction they could offer students, it could be useful to alter the training ward experience to a more collaborative problem-solving approach. Here students could jointly plan their work, undertake it, evaluate it and then reflect upon it.
- Participation in team duties on the training ward has been problematic. To overcome this difficulty, students could be set fixed times during their shifts for when they jointly participate in team duties and for when they undertake profession-specific duties.
- To overcome the difficulty of students being able to cope with both profession-specific and teamworking roles on the training ward, it may be beneficial to alter the experience to emphasise the inter-professional nature of this placement. Therefore the training ward would be regarded as the inter-professional ward placement, unlike the students' more traditional profession-specific placements.
- Maintaining a mix of suitable patients for the training ward and obtaining informed consent proved time consuming and largely fell to senior nurses. Mechanisms for easing this burden should be considered.

This inter-professional initiative has the potential to develop into a valuable, mature project that provides an innovative educational experience for students, and staff development opportunities that are unique in the UK. Such a beacon has the potential to improve recruitment and retention in the associated trusts and schools. Therefore, the training ward should recommence, modified in the light of experience gained from the pilot. In addition, in order to develop a robust, comprehensive understanding of this

ward and its effects on students, staff and patients, a continuing
evaluation needs to be part of this initiative.

Glossary

M-Student	Medical Student
N-Facilitator	Nurse Facilitator
N-Student	Nursing Student
OT	Occupational Therapy
PBL	Problem-Based Learning
P-Facilitator	Profession-Specific Facilitator
PT	Physiotherapy

Acknowledgements

The evaluation of the training ward pilot was funded by the
Special Trustees of St Bartholomew's Hospital.

The staff, students and evaluators of the training ward in
Linköping were generous with their time and advice during the
development of the London inter-professional training ward.
This has been a fine example of international, inter-professional
collaboration that is likely to spawn further educational development and evaluation in both countries.

Finally, our appreciation goes to all the patients, students and
staff who contributed to the training ward pilot project.

References

Bloomfield, D (1997) *Actuarial Examinations: What Can be Learnt From
the Students' Perspective?*, unpublished PhD Thesis, Institute of
Education, University of London.
Carpenter, J (1995) Implementing community care. In Soothill, K,
Mackay, L and Webb, C (eds), *Interprofessional Relations in Health
Care*. London: Edward Arnold.
Casto, M (1994) Interprofessional work in the USA – education and
practice. In Leathard, A (ed.), Going Interprofessional: Working
Together for Health and Welfare. London: Routledge.

Dacre, J and Nicol, M (1996) *The Clinical Skills Matrix*. Oxford: Radcliffe Medical Press.

Department of Health (1998) A First Class Service: Quality in the NHS. London: HMSO.

Dienst, E and Byl, N (1981) Evaluation of an educational program in health care teams, *Journal of Community Health*, **6**, 282–98.

Elywin, G, Rapport, F and Kinnersley, P (1998) Primary health care teams re-engineered, *Journal of Interprofessional Care*, **12**, 189–98.

Entwistle, N (1987) A model of the teaching-learning process. In Richardson, J, Eysenck, M and Piper, D (eds), *Student Learning: Research in Education and Cognitive Psychology*. Milton Keynes: SRHE and OUP.

Fallsberg, M and Wijma, K (1999) Student attitudes towards the goals of an interprofessional training ward, *Medical Teacher* **21**, 576–81.

Freeth, D and Nicol, M (1998) Learning clinical skills: an interprofessional approach, *Nurse Education Today*, **18**, 455–61.

Freeth, D and Reeves, S (1999) *Interprofessional Training Ward Pilot Phase: Evaluation Project Report*. Internal Research Report No. 14, London: St Bartholomew School of Nursing and Midwifery, City University (ISBN 1900804 12 3).

Funnell, P (1995) Exploring the value of interprofessional shared learning, In Soothill, K, Mackay, L and Webb, C (eds), *Interprofessional Relations in Health Care*. London: Edward Arnold.

Headrick, L, Wilcock, P and Batalden, P (1998) Interprofessional working and continuing medical education, *British Medical Journal*, **316**, 771–4.

Howkins, E and Allison, A (1997) Shared learning for primary health teams: a success story, *Nurse Education Today*, **17**, 225–31.

Hughes, L and Lucas, J (1997) An evaluation of problem based learning in the multiprofessional education curriculum for the health professions, *Journal of Interprofessional Care*, **11**, 77–88.

Itano, J, Williams, J, Deaton, M and Oishi, N (1991) Impact of a student interdisciplinary oncology team project. *Journal of Cancer Education*, **6**, 219–26.

Jaques, D (1984) *Learning in Groups*. Beckenham: Croom Helm.

Knowles, M (1990) *The Adult Learner: A Neglected Species*. (4th edn), Houston: Gulf.

McGrath, J (1990) Time matters in groups. In Galegher, J, Kraut, R and Egido, C (eds), *Intellectual Teamwork*. New Jersey: Lawrence Erlbaum.

Miller, C, Ross, N and Freeman, M (1999) *Shared Learning and Clinical Teamwork: New Directions in Education for Multiprofessional Practice*. London: ENB.

Morgan, A (1993) *Improving your Students' Learning: Reflections on the Experience of Study*. London: Kogan Page.

Parsell, G, Spalding, R and Bligh, J (1998) Shared Goals, shared learning: evaluation of a multiprofessional course for undergraduate students, *Medical Education*, **32**, 304–11.

Pietroni, P (1991) Stereotypes or archetypes? A study of perceptions amongst health care students, *Journal of Interprofessional Care*, **5**, 61–9.

Pirrie, A, Elsegood, J and Hall, J (1998) *Evaluating Multidisciplinary Education in Health Care*. Final Report of a 24-month funded study, London: Department of Health.

Reeves, S and Pryce, A (1998) Emerging themes: an exploratory research project of an interprofessional module for medical, dental and nursing students, *Nurse Education Today*, **18**, 534–41.

Rogers, C (1969) *Freedom to Learn*. Columbus, ohio: Merril.

Sandén, I and Wahlström, O (1996) *Training Ward 30*. Sweden: Linköping University.

Snadden, D and Bain, J (1998) Hospital doctors, general practitioners and dentists learning together, *Medical Education*, **32**, 376–83.

Studdy, S, Nicol, M and Fox-Hiley, A (1994) Teaching and learning clinical skills, part 1 – development of a multidisciplinary skills centre, *Nurse Education Today*, **14**, 177–85.

Thomas, M (1995) Learning to be a better team player: initiatives in continuing education in primary health care. In Soothill, K, Mackay, L and Webb, C (eds), *Interprofessional Relations in Health Care*. London: Edward Arnold.

Wahlström, O and Sandén, I (1998) Multiprofessional training ward at Linköping University: early experience, *Education for Health*, **11**, 225–31.

West, M (1997) A failure of function: teamwork in primary health care, *Journal of Interprofessional Care*, **11**(2), 205–16.

Zwarenstein, M, Atkins, J, Barr, H, Hammick, M, Koppel, I and Reeves, S (1999) A systematic review of interprofessional education, *Journal of Interprofessional Care*, **13**, 417–24.

8

Inter-professional Education: the Way Forward

Sally Glen

Introduction

Preceding chapters in this book provide examples of inter-professional education. Inter-professional initiatives have been increasing over the past five years. This increase in inter-professional initiatives has been in response to increasing calls from successive governments for health and social care professionals to work more closely together for the benefit of the users of health and social care services. The importance of an inter-professional approach to health and social care is emphasised in which all the professionals who contribute to the care of a user work not just alongside each other but also inter-professionally, as a team. The aim is to provide a 'seamless service' for users. This means that they can move between hospital and community without gaps or stumbling blocks in communication about their needs; that the different people caring for them, whether in hospital or at home, are well informed about what other carers' interventions have been; and that there is an agreed plan for their future care. However, whilst moves towards integrated programmes for health and social care professionals are undoubtedly in evidence, the objectives are often not always made explicit (see Chapters 1 and 2).

Policy documents often remain silent in terms of suggesting a strategy of how inter-professional education might be implemented. For Loxley (1997: 72) this is the reason why the inter-professional education 'remains a largely haphazard and localised activity'. The various stakeholders involved also see the advantages and disadvantages of enhancing inter-professional work and under-pinning it with inter-professional learning from their own per-spectives and within the context of their own organisational, financial and professional constraints (Miller, 1999). This issue is explored in the following section.

Multiple stakeholder perspectives

Some of the factors contributing to current consideration of the role of inter-professional teamwork in health and social care, such as continuity of care for users, role blurring and skill mix, are different from those preoccupying managers of educational provision in the education institutions, such as greater flexibility of course provision to a wider field of students. Given the poten-tial for differences in the driving forces behind shared learning initiatives and the rapid rate of change in both sectors, the devel-opments in the service could become out of tune with those in education. As Miller (1999: 2) notes, 'From the student's point of view, a new kind of theory practice gap could be created between the reality of multi-professional teamwork in different types of teams and shared learning education.' Evidence from Miller's report (ENB, 1999) suggests that this is happening. This research report suggests that the 'common context' approach is a major missed opportunity for addressing shared learning in a way that will feed into inter-professional practice.

There is also a fundamental danger. Emphasis upon common learning needs can be at the expense of special learning needs, specialist learning made more necessary by the exponential growth in medical knowledge and technological advance leading to more specialities and sub-specialities in medicine and hence in related professions. A new starting point is an education route which looks towards inter-professional practice and the benefits to users from collaborative practice for inspiration about teaching content and learning methods. By setting up learning experiences for students which address the processes and problems of inter-professional working, shared learning which benefits practice will come closer (Miller *et al.*, 2001). The arguments for 'common learning' are still valid where unnecessary repetition of teaching is avoided and the viability of small cohorts is assured. The dilemma for education appears to be:

- either a move towards a possible core curriculum which has the possible advantage of economics of scale, but has little value-added context
- and/or a closer look at service needs and select those areas of the curriculum that support the development of teams around shared professional agendas.

Miller *et al.*'s (1999) research suggests that, for inter-professional learning to occur there is a strong argument for reconceptualising what could be achieved if it is to enhance professionals' ability to work together. There is no doubt that a more integrated approach to the preparation of learners needs to be knowledgeable and reflective, responsive and skilful practitioners is required.

An integrated approach to care

To facilitate the development of an integrated approach to the preparation of learners to be knowledgeable, reflective, responsive and skilled practitioners, it may be necessary to dismantle some of the protective fences which have served to sustain professional apartheid. More importantly, however, it is essential that conditions are created which can foster co-operation, collaboration and the development of productive partnerships. In considering how best to achieve an integrated approach to the preparation of practitioners, it is necessary to try to envisage the desired end point. Effective care requires an approach which does not restrict practitioners to a traditional range of activities. It involves the development of new organisations and networks to work in new ways to establish a new pattern of services (see Chapter 3).

There is a need to move away from models of professional and vocational education which seek to prepare students for particular jobs in particular organisations and towards an approach which promotes flexibility and adaptability. It is essential that the practitioners of the future who wish to specialise in caring for

a particular client group (for example, people with learning disabilities and their families; people with mental health problems,
or older adults) are able to pursue a career which will entail cross-
ing and re-crossing organisational and sectoral boundaries. In its
consultation document the Department of Health (2000) suggests
that it wants to look at the workforce in a new way, 'as teams of
people rather than different tribes'. This report emphasises the
need for teamwork and flexible working to make the best use
of skills. Barriers between occupational groups should be done
away with and more flexible careers opened up to maximise the
contribution of all to patient care. Education and training should
be modernised to equip staff to work in a complex and changing
NHS. It will thus be of advantage if the practitioner is able to
work effectively with different client groups – both within the
context of the NHS and in relation to other types of services. In
addition, it will be necessary to ensure that people are able to
make smooth transitions between service provision, development,
management and planning. In examining how best to ensure
flexibility and adaptability, it is necessary to take into account the
requirements of both new students and existing practitioners
whose knowledge, skills and attitude may no longer suit the
requirements of particular services. The document suggests that
the relationship between the NHS and providers of education
and training neds to be improved. It finds 'a disfunction between
the needs of the NHS and the desires of education providers',
with 'an over-academisation of training'. Selection is liable to
emphasise academic ability over caring skills. Higher education
is said to value research more than teaching as an indicator of
success. Some lecturers, says the report, are out of touch with
modern service needs which, as a result, are not picked up in
revising curricula (Barr, 2000). The DOH Document 'Investment
and Reform for NHS Staff: Taking Forward The NHS Plan (DOH
2001)' reiterates the Labour government's committment to developing and introducing common learning programmes for all
health professionals, based on core skills, designed on a more
flexible basis and providing easier routes and opportunities for
individuals to transfer between education and training programmes
and maximise future career pathways. The government also wants
to see students learning together in clinical practice placements –
the joint ENB/DH booke 1 (2001) 'Placements in Focus' stresses

that where possible placements should be multi-professional so that students can see how all staff contribute to patient care.

Several regulatory bodies already require students to demonstrate skills in collaborative working before they can qualify for their respective professions; see, for example, nursing (UKCC, 1989), social work (CCETSW, 1995) and medicine (GMC, 1996). Account needs also to be taken of the framework for higher education qualifications being developed by the Quality Assurance Agency (QAA, 2000). Subject benchmarks will provide the conceptual framework that gives each discipline coherence and identity. It remains to be seen how these will frame commonalities not only between academic disciplines but also practice professions. Implications for boundary definition and for professional and inter-professional education and practice could be far reaching, working relations being forged between the QAA, professional and regulatory bodies and the NHS will become even more important.

The challenge facing educators, confederations and validating bodies is how to create coherent programmes which can enable both new entrants and existing practitioners who are undertaking further study to exit with academically appropriate and vocationally relevant qualifications that adequately reflect their capabilities and competencies. What appears to be lacking is an integrated approach to funding, approval and accreditation which can both ensure that standards are maintained and encourages innovation.

A system sympathetic to innovation

A system is required at regional or confederation level that is sympathetic to innovation. Such a system would:

- have an understanding of the range of funding resources, preferably with a guide to explaining how the system can be used to the best advantage
- recognise the structures involved and the people who manage them
- have an ethos that responds helpfully to bottom-up innovations
- involve champions and advocates – people of influence who can rise above the tribalism

- help people to become more expert in the art of putting education packages together; the barriers are often not structural but
  tribal and can be overcome by local advocates and the dissemination of good practice – why are some initiatives successful
  when the efforts of others are not?

Many of the issues related to education barriers are also sociolo-
gical rather than structural. We are in a multi-professional rather
than an inter-professional world and this has advantages and
disadvantages. The skills needed to overcome barriers are those
of developing, maturing, sustaining and maintaining relationships –
relationships which need to be continuous, not episodic (Chapters 4, 5 and 6). Inter-dependency goes hand-in-hand with some
loss of organisational autonomy, and can mean loss of power
to define your own agenda, loss of control over some of your
resources and loss of loyalty. The importance of personal relationships in collaborative ventures is important. There needs to
be more recognition of the important role played by key people
who have the social, political and professional skills to move easily between organisations and professions, moving up and down
administrative structures and providing the grease that makes
the collaboration wheel run that much more easily. Developing
inter-professional education undoubtedly requires extraordinary
organisation and managerial skill, and it cannot become a reality
without institutional and inter-institutional commitments. Current education and training reforms contain seeds of tension.
Developing flexible working and collaborative practice may seem
to be one and the same, but pursuit of the former may be at the
expense of the latter. If the pace of change generates resistance
and tension between agencies and between professions, inter-
professional education can help to alleviate such tension – but
only help. It can complement consultation between the parties,
but is no substitute. As conceived, inter-professional education
encouraged collaboration between more or less stable organisational groups. It must do so now between groups whose roles
and responsibilities are subject to review as power shifts and
boundaries are redrawn. Inter-professioal education is called upon
to reconcile objectives that may be in conflict, affecting changes
in service delivery, modifying the workforce and encouraging
collaboration in the interests of service users. Its role becomes

more complex and more difficult, but also more important, as an agent of change (Barr, 2000).

Finally, there is the need to find evidence of the link between the positive outcomes of inter-professional education for learners and the potential for the enhancement of inter-professional working.

An evidence-based agenda

Within the context of evidence and practice, inter-professional education is not easily identifiable as good (Barr, Clague and Hammick, 1999a). Ongoing work from two systematic reviews of inter-professional education (Zwarenstein *et al.*, 1999, Barr *et al.*, 1999b). Evaluations of inter-professional education remain few and uneven in quality (Barr and Shaw, 1995; Barr *et al.*, 2000; Koppel *et al.*, 2001). An inter-professional education joint evaluation team (JET) was convened to conduct systematic reviews of evaluations of inter-professional education. Research of the kind that JET is doing serves four purposes. It establishes:

1. what is known already
2. the means by which it has become known
3. questions remaining to be addressed in prospective research
4. ways in which research methodology can be improved.

Of the outcomes reported by JET, the most telling highlights differences in relation to locations. Positive outcomes reported from evaluations of inter-professional education based in higher education were overwhelmingly in the form of reactions to the learning experiences, changes in attitude or perception, and the acquisition of knowledge and/or skills. Positive outcomes reported from work-based inter-professional education also included changes in the organisation of practice and effects in patient or clients. This difference may reinforce assertions that inter-professional education is only effective when it is work based, but like is not being compared with like: university-based and work-based inter-professional education must be seen as different but complementary, each capable of reinforcing the other.

Finally, there has been much written about new inter-professional collaborations, rather less about established or terminated collaborations Freeth (2001) using 'The Clinical Skills Initiative' at St Bartholomew's School of Nursing and Midwifery, City University, as a case study of a sustained collaboration. She argues that a combination of continued need to collaborate and empowerment to do so, creates favourable conditions for sustained collaboration.

Conclusion

If inter-professional education is to become a reality, innovative new approaches are required. The models of education and curriculum we currently have will not be able to meet the evolving service requirements of the future. Workforce planning requirements will need to take cognisance of the increasing need for practitioners to be able to operate effectively in both primary and secondary health and social care settings and to be truly able to deliver 'seamless care'. Major reviews will be necessary over the next few years within pre-registration and continuing professional development programmes to allow for learning opportunities across nursing, midwifery, medicine, dentistry, social work and the professions allied to medicine.

References

Barr, H (2000) *Inter-professional Education 1997–2000, Centre for the Advancement of Inter-professional Education.* Report commissioned by the UKCC.

Barr, H and Shaw, L (1995) *Shared Learning: Selected examples from the literature.* London: CAIPE.

Barr, H, Clague, B and Hammick, M (1999a) Evaluation of the Effectiveness of Interprofessional Education, English National Board Conference, November 24, London.

Barr, H, Freeth, D, Hammick, M, Koppel, I and Reeves, S (2000) *Establishing the Evidence Base for Interprofessional Education: Outcomes from three reviews by the Joint Evaluation Team.* CAIPE Bulletin Number 18, Summer.

Barr, H, Hammick, M, Koppel, I and Reeves, S (1999b) Evaluating Inter-professional Education: Two Systematic Reviews for Health and Social Care, *British Educational Research Journal*, **25**, 533–43.

CCETSW (1995) *Assuring Quality in the Diploma in Social Work – 1, Rules and Requirements for the Dip SW London*. Central Council for Education and Training in Social Work.

Department of Health (2000) *A Health Service of Talents: Developing The NHS Workforce*. London: HMSO.

Department of Health (2001) *Investment and Reform for NHS Staff: Taking Forward the NHS Plan*. London: HMSO.

ENB (English National Board for Nursing, Midwifery and Health Visiting) (1999) *The Role of Collaborative/Shared Learning in Pre- and Post Registration Education in Nursing, Midwifery and Health Visiting*. London: ENB.

English National Board for Nursing, Midwifery and Health Visiting and Department of Health (2001) *Placements in Focus*, London: ENB.

Freeth, D (2001) Sustaining Inter-professional Collaboration, *Journal of Inter-professional Care*, **15**(1), 37–46.

GMC (1996) *Recommendations on General Clinical Training*. London: General Medical Council.

Koppel, I, Barr, H, Reeves, S, Freeth, S and Hammick, M (2001) Establishing a Systematic Approach to Evaluating the Effectiveness of Interprofessional Education Issues in *Inter-disciplinary Care*, **3**(1), January 41–9.

Loxley, A (1997) *Collaboration in Health and Welfare: Working with Difference*. London: Jessica Kingsley.

Miller, C (1999) Shared Learning for Pre-Qualification Health and Social Care Students; Have the Universities Missed the Point?, BERA Conference, 3 September, University of Sussex.

Miller, C, Freeman, Mond Ross, N (2001) *Interprofessional Practice in Health and Social Care: Challenging to Shared Learning Agenda*. London: Arnold.

QAA (2000) *Draft Handbook for Academic Review*. Gloucester Quality Assurance Agency.

UKCC (1989) *Project 2000: Rule 18 Statutory Instrument*. No. 1456, London: United Kingdom, Central Council for Nursing, Midwifery and Health Visiting.

Zwarenstein, M, Atkins, J, Hammick, M, Barr, H, Koppel, I and Reeves, S (1999) Interprofessional Education and Systematics Review: A New Initiative in Evaluation, *Journal of Interprofessional Care*, **13**(4), 417–24.

Index

Allen, D.   17
Areskog, N. H.   64
Atkinson, P.   9

Banta, D. and Fox, R.   15, 16
Barclay Report (1982)   28
Barnett, R.   10
Barr, H.   7, 27
Barrows, H. S.   68
Barts   *see* St Bartholomew
  (London)
Baxter, C.   30
Beattie, A.   10, 18–19
Bernstein, B.   9
*Better Services for the Mentally
  Handicapped* (1971)   42
Briggs Report (1972)   42
Brown, T. M.   15
Butler-Sloss Report (1988)   26

CAIPE   *see* Centre for the
  Advancement of
  Interprofessional
  Education in Primary Care and
  Community Care
Calman, K.   29
Caring for People in the Community
  (White Paper) (1989)   28
Carpenter, J.   12
Casto, R. M. and Julie, M. C.   101
CCETSW   *see* Central Council
  for Education and
  Training in Social Work
Central Council for Education
  and Training in Social
  Work (CCETSW)   43, 45, 46,
  47, 48, 50, 51, 54

Centre for the Advancement
  of Interprofessional
  Education in Primary
  Care and Community Care
  (CAIPE)   35
Certificate in Social Service
  (CSS)   43
Cherasky, M.   35
Child Abuse in Cleveland
  report (1988)   26
City University (London)   116, 117
Clinical Skills Initiative   146;
  advantages/disadvantages   87;
  aims   85; and clinical
  governance   92–5;
  discussion/evaluation   91–2;
  patient scenario example   88;
  programme   86–7;
  structure   87–91
clinical/midwifery students joint
  programme   *see* normal labour
  teaching programme
Clyde Report (1992)   4–5
Coit Butler, F.   7
Common Competency
  Framework   47, 48–50
computer assisted learning (CAL)
  programme   63, 66, 68, 74
Consulting, J. M.   29
Core Competencies   *see* Common
  Competency Framework
Creating Lifelong Learners   47
Cribb, A. and Bignold, S.   11

Day,   30
Department of Health
  (DOH)   28, 29, 142

Dienst, E. and Byl, N.   125
Dingwall, R. and McIntosh, J.   16
Diploma in Social Care
   (DipSW)   47

education, and aims of
   inter-disciplinarity   10–11;
   changes in   2–3;
   delivery/evaluation of   12–15;
   and employment   8;
   and integrated curriculum
   9–12; as multi-disciplinary/
   modular   8–9;
   multi-professionalism in   7–15;
   professional/higher   7–8, 9
EMPE   *see* European Network
   for Development of
   Multi-professional
   Education in Health
   Sciences
ENB   *see* English National Board
   for Nursing, Midwifery and
   Health Visiting
English National Board for
   Nursing, Midwifery and
   Health Visiting (ENB)
   45, 47, 48
ethics, shared teaching in,
   aims/learning outcomes
   102–3; arguments for   98;
   background   97–8;
   classroom availability   107;
   collaboration meeting
   points   106–7; educational
   strategy   104; evaluation   110;
   facilitator availability   107–8;
   ideal of   98–101;
   intermediate level   102–3,
   114–15; junior level   102,
   112–14; learning/teaching
   tools   105–6; management
   of student numbers   103;
   pilot study   100–1;

progress to date   110;
   reality challenges   106–9;
   sample case studies/statements
   105; seminar format   99;
   senior level   103, 115;
   staff development   109;
   student knowledge base   108–9;
   students' evaluation of
   sessions   112–15;
   and teamwork   99–100
European Network for
   Development of
   Multi-professional
   Education in Health
   Sciences (EMPE)   35
Exeter University   34

facilitators, and burn-out   133;
   nurse-facilitators   121–2;
   and PBL/reflection
   distinction   124;
   positive attitude of   132;
   profession-specific   121;
   value of   124
Fife College of Health Studies   62
Frederick, C.   33
Freeth, D.   146;
   and Nicol, M.   13
Friedson, E.   13

General Nursing Council   43

Harden, R. M.   13, 33
Harvey, L. *et al*   8
Hawthorne effect   133
Headrick, L. *et al*   16
'Health for All by the Year 2000'
   initiative   2
health policies, and clinical
   conflict   5–6; and curbing
   of freedom/autonomy of
   clinicians   6; and integration
   of health/social services   3, 5;

health policies – *continued*
    partnership aspect 6–7;
    three-tier strategy 3
health practice, biographical
    model 18; biotechnical
    model 18; communitarian
    model 18; ecological
    model 18; relationships
    in 16–19;
    teams/teamworking 15–16
Hearn, J. 30
holistic approach 40, 44
Holm, S. 100, 105
Horder, J. 27, 76
hospital closures 42, 43, 44
Howard, J. and Byl, N. 12
Hurst, K. 8, 19

integrated, care 3, 5, 6, 41,
    46, 141–3; curriculum 9
inter-professional,
    collaboration 12;
    initiatives 35; integration 2;
    practitioner/user effects 31–2;
    relationships 31–2, 102–3
inter-professional education 15,
    26–7, 84; benefits of 139;
    defined 86; evidence-based
    agenda 145–6;
    as haphazard/localised
    activity 139–40;
    initiatives 139; and
    innovation 143–5; and
    integrated care 141–3;
    multiple stakeholder
    perspectives 140–1
inter-professional training
    ward, background 116;
    described 117–18;
    discussion of findings 119–33;
    evaluation of 118–19;
    facilitation 121–2; future
    development 134–6;

Hawthorne effect 133; impact
    on service delivery 131–3;
    learning/teaching aspects 121–5;
    off-ward learning 123–4;
    problem-based
    approach 126–7; real life
    experience 120–1; strengths
    of pilot scheme 133–4; student
    learning objectives 124–5;
    student support 122–3;
    team duties 127–9;
    thematic presentation 119–20;
    training ward patients 129–31;
    two-week placement 125
'Investment and Reform for
    NHS Staff' (2001) 142

Jacques, D. 125
Jay Report (1979) 42–3
Johnston, K. 9
joint evaluation team (JET) 145
joint training 41–2; application
    of lessons learned 58–9;
    assessment of programme
    50–1; based on partnership
    50–1; challenges encountered
    51–3; common foundation
    programme (CFP) 45–6, 56;
    competency-based approach
    40; evaluation of South Bank
    programme 55–8; framework
    of common competencies 47;
    historical context 42–3; and
    inter-professional competence
    48–50; lessons learned from
    previous programmes 54–5;
    local demand for 43–4;
    programme evaluation 53–4;
    programmes for 41; rationale
    for 44–5; structure of
    programme 45–6; value of
    integrated/holistic
    approach 40–1

King's Fund partnership
  Trust 101
knowledge/skills 144, 145;
  generic/profession-specific
  29; sharing of 88–9;
  wider/varied 58

labour, midwifery/clinical
  students programme *see*
  normal labour teaching
  programme
learning disabilities, joint training
  for *see* joint training
learning disability nurse,
  qualifications xiv, 43
Leathard, A. 1, 2
Leiba, T. 30
London NHS Trust 117
London University 116
Loxley, A. 5, 13, 139

McGrath, J. 125
Mackay, L. 16; *et al* 6, 98
McKiel, R. E. *et al* 98, 101
Marylebone Centre trust 34
Mason, E. J. and
  Parascondola, J. 12
Mazur, H. *et al* 12
medical model 54
Melia, K. 9
mental disability 30; training for
  see joint training
midwifery/clinical students
  joint programme
  see normal labour teaching
  programme
Miller, C. 140; *et al* 15, 141
Millerson, G. 8
Modernising Social Services
  (1998) 41
Montefore Hospital (USA) 35
Moray Institute (Edinburgh) 12
Morris, P. 42

multi-professional education,
  assumptions 29–32; benefits
  of 36, 61; curriculum
  co-ordination 63–4, 85; and
  employment 7–12; and the
  future 34–6; in health
  care 12–15; initiatives 34–6;
  introduction of 61–2; need
  for 25–6; opportunities
  for 28–9; and pre-registration
  courses 27; provision of 36;
  research/practice tension 27;
  and seamless service 28, 139;
  terminology 26–8;
  theories 32–4
multi-professionalism,
  defined 1–2, 20; in
  education 7–15; introduction
  of 19; in policy 2–7, 139;
  in practice 15–19

National Health Service
  Executive 28
National Health Service
  (NHS) 41, 44, 142, 143
The New NHS Modern, Dependable
  (1997) 6, 29, 41
normal labour teaching
  programme, and attitude
  questionnaire 71–3, 82–3;
  background 61–4;
  and clinical skills 68–9;
  coincidence of timetables
  63–4; creation of CAL
  package 63; delivery of 67–9;
  evaluation process 70–1;
  evaluation results 71–4;
  expansion of 76;
  implementation 64–71;
  implications for the future 76;
  initiative for 64–5, 76–7;
  and integrated boards 69;
  keys to success of 75;

normal labour teaching – *continued*
and knowledge
questionnaire   71;
limitations of   74–5;
midwifery/obstetrics
relationship   63; planning
of   67; and problem-based
learning   68; sample
integrated teaching
boards   78–81;
teaching/learning
methods   65–6

obstetricians   *see* normal labour
teaching programme
occupational therapy (OT)
students   118, 135
Ohio Interprofessional
Commission   35–6
Ovretveit, P. *et al*   1, 31

Parsell, G. and Bligh, J.   27, 76;
et al   13
partnerships   7, 41; assessment
panel   50–1; authorities/
agencies   28; management
committee   50;
as productive   141
patients   14; and clinical
skills initiative   88;
and inter-professional training
ward participation   118,
119, 129–31, 134;
relationship with
professionals   31–2
Peckham Experiment   35
Peter, E. and Gallop, R.   99–100
physical disability   30
physiotherapy (PT)
students   118, 135
Pioneer Health Centre
(London)   35
Pirrie, A. *et al*   26, 27, 32

'Placements in Focus'
(2001)   142–3; social
work   143
Platt, L. J.   98
practitioner relationships   31–2
pre-/post-registration   3, 61, 85
primary care groups   41
problem-based learning (PBL),
in inter-professional
teaching   65–6, 67–8, 74;
in training ward   118, 121,
124, 126–7, 135
professional/user
relationship   31–2

Quality Assurance Agency
(QCA)   143
Queen Mary and Westfield
College (QMW)
(London)   116, 117

race/ethnicity issues   30–1
reflective practice   19
regulation   29
Rodgers, J.   98
role-shadowing   129

St Bartholomew (Bart's)   116, 117
St Bartholomew School of
Nursing and Midwifery
(London)   116, 117
Schon, D. A.   33
School of Medicine and Dentistry
see University of Dundee
School of Nursing and
Midwifery   *see* University
of Dundee
sex/gender issues   30
social model   54
social services, joint training
programme   *see* joint
training
Social Services Directorate   28

South Bank University 34; evaluation of programme 55–8; joint training programme 43, 45–53
Spencer, M. H. 32
Svensson, R. 16
Szasz, G. 12, 33

Tayside College Nursing and Midwifery 62
teams, teamwork 29, 35–6, 140, 142; duties 127–9; and mental handicap 43; participants 118; reflection sessions 123–4
The Royal London School of Medicine and Dentistry 116
Thomas, M. 121
Tope, R. 2, 13
Tower Hamlets Health Care Trust 117

University of Bobigny (Paris Nord) 35
University of Dundee 61, 62; Clinical Skills Initiative 86–95; normal labour teaching programme 61–77; shared teaching in ethics 97–110
University of East London 117
University of Limburg (Maastricht) 35
University of Linkoping (Sweden) 34, 35, 117
University of Westminster 34–5
user/professional relationship 31–2

ward placement *see* inter-professional training ward
West, M. 15, 20
Wicks, D. 18
Working for Patients, Education and Training (1989) 28
'Working Together: teamwork' (1994) 29
World Health Organisation (WHO) 2–3, 26, 100

zones of practice 33